Air Fryer for Beginners

A Cooking Guide for Getting Delicious Meals out of your New Air Fryer

By Samantha Hendrick

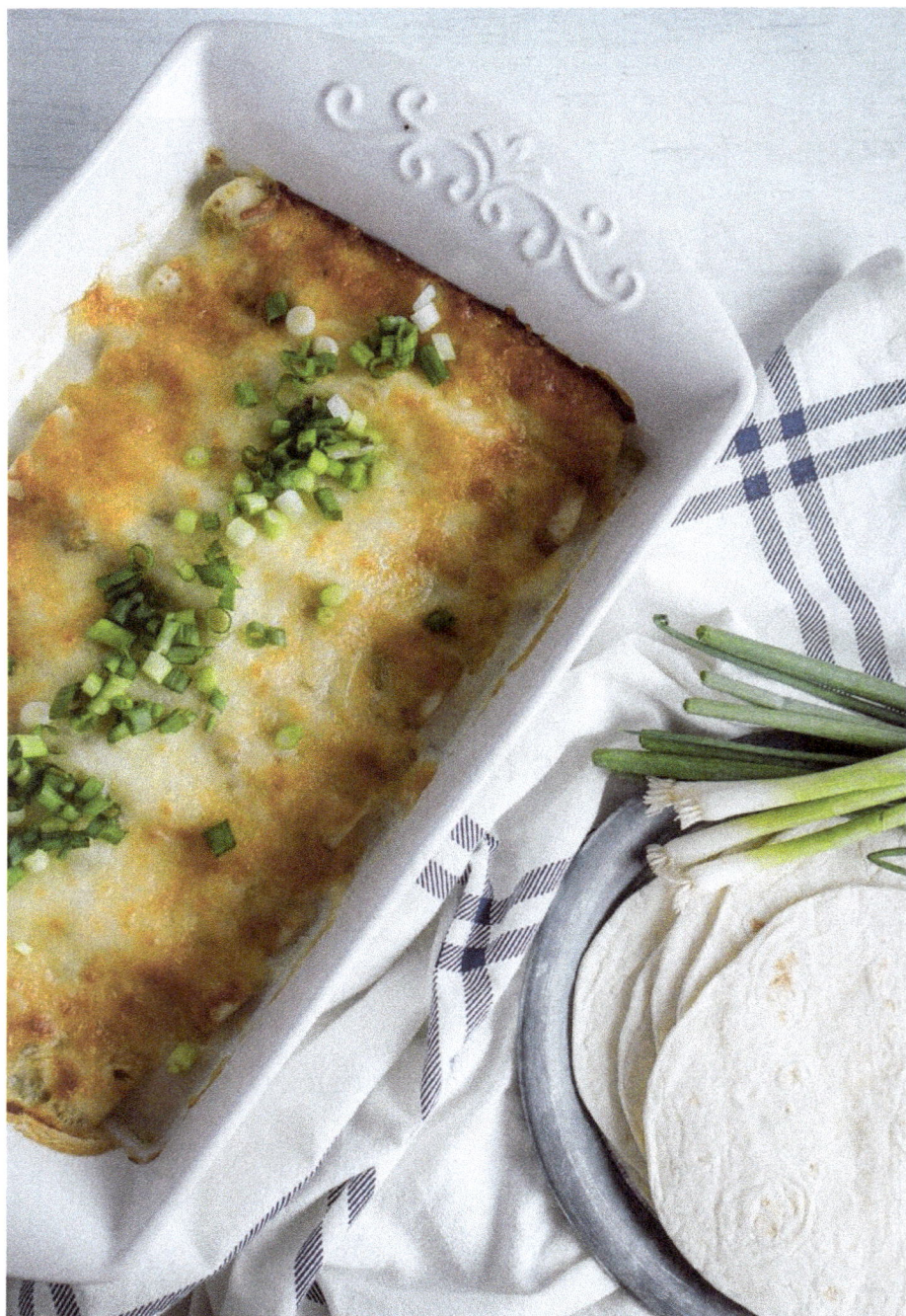

The content within this book has been derived from various sources. Please consult a licensed professional before attempting any techniques outlined in this book.

By reading this document, the reader agrees that under no circumstances is the author responsible for any losses, direct or indirect, which are incurred as a result of the use of information contained within this document, including, but not limited to, — errors, omissions, or inaccuracies.

Table of Contents

Cajun Spiced Veggie-Shrimp Bake

Servings per Recipe: 4

Cooking Time: 20 minutes

Ingredients:

- 1 Bag of Frozen Mixed Vegetables
- 1 Tbsp Gluten-Free Cajun Seasoning /15g
- Olive Oil Spray
- Season with salt and pepper
- Small Shrimp Peeled & Deveined (Regular Size Bag about 50-80 Small Shrimp)

Instructions:

1) With a cooking spray lightly grease a baking pan with any oil of your choice. Add all ingredients to the baking pan and stir well to coat. Season with pepper and salt to taste.
2) Cook on 3300 F or 166°C for 10 minutes. Stir after every 5 minutes.
3) Serve and enjoy.

Nutrition Information:

- Calories per Serving: 78
- Carbs: 13.2g
- Protein: 2.8g
- Fat: 1.5g

Celery leaves 'n Garlic-oil Grilled Turbot

Servings per Recipe: 2

Cooking Time: 20 minutes

Ingredients:

- ½ cup chopped celery leaves /65g
- 1 clove of garlic, minced
- 2 tablespoons olive oil /30ml
- 2 whole turbot, scaled and head removed
- Salt and pepper to taste

Instructions:

1) Preheat the air fryer to 3900 F or 199°C using the air fryer settings.
2) Place the grill pan in the air fryer.
3) Season the turbot with salt, pepper, garlic, celery leaves and then brush with oil.
4) Gently place in the grill pan and cook for 20 minutes until the fish becomes flaky

Nutrition information:

- Calories per serving: 269
- Carbs: 3.3g
- Protein: 66.2g
- Fat: 25.6g

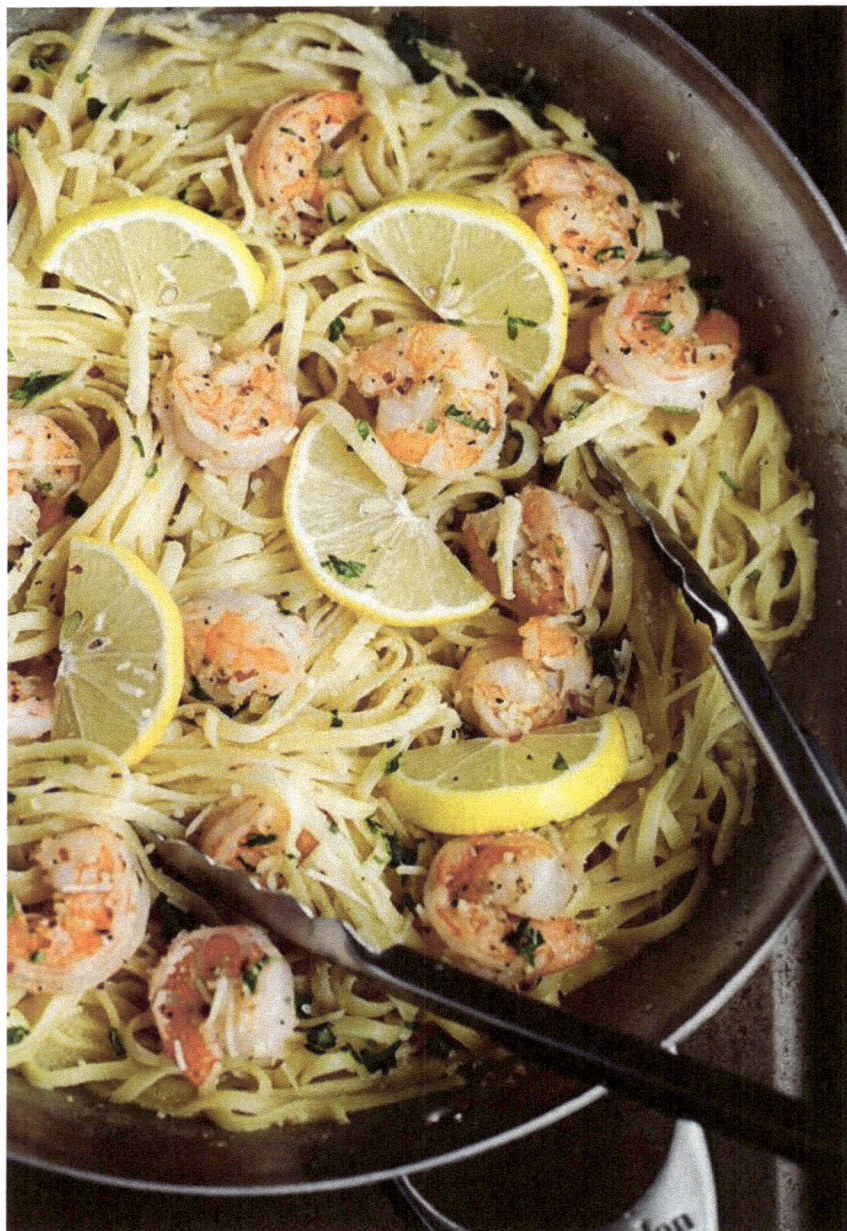

Char-Grilled Drunken Halibut

Servings per Recipe: 6

Cooking Time: 20 minutes

Ingredients:

- 1 tablespoon chili powder /15g
- 2 cloves of garlic, minced
- 3 pounds halibut fillet, skin removed /1350g
- 4 tablespoons dry white wine /60g
- 4 tablespoons olive oil /60ml
- Salt and pepper to taste

Instructions:

1) Put all ingredients in the large Ziploc bag.
2) Place in the fridge and allow to marinate for 2 hours.
3) Preheat the air fryer to 3900 F or 199°C .
4) Place the grill pan accessory in the air fryer.
5) Grill the fish for 20 minutes making sure to turn it over every 5 minutes.

Nutrition information:

- Calories per serving: 385
- Carbs: 1.7g
- Protein: 33g
- Fat: 40.6g

Clams with Herbed Butter in Packets

Servings per Recipe: 2

Cooking Time: 20 Minutes

Ingredients:

- ½ cup unsalted butter, diced /65g
- 1 tablespoon dill, chopped /15g
- 1 tablespoon fresh freshly squeezed lemon juice/15ml
- 1 tablespoon parsley, chopped /15g
- 24 littleneck clams, scrubbed clean
- Lemon wedges
- Salt and pepper to taste

Instructions:

1) Preheat mid-air fryer to 3900 F or 199°C .
2) Place the grill pan in the air fryer.
3) Place clams and other ingredients on a large foil. Fold the foil and wrap the edges.
4) Place on the grill pan and cook for 15 to 20 minutes or until all clams are opened.

Nutrition information:

- Calories per serving: 384
- Carbs: 6g
- Protein: 18g

- Fat: 32g

Cocktail Prawns in Air Fryer

Servings per Recipe: 1

Cooking Time: 8 minutes

Ingredients:

- ½ teaspoon black pepper /2.5g
- ½ teaspoon sea salt /2.5g
- 1 tablespoon ketchup /15ml
- 1 tablespoon white wine vinegar /15ml
- 1 teaspoon chili flakes /5g
- 1 teaspoon chili powder /5g
- 12 prawns, shelled and deveined

Instructions:

1) Preheat the air fryer to 390 0 F or 199°C .
2) Place the shrimps in a bowl.
3) Stir in the other ingredients in a bowl. Coat shrimps with the content of the bowl.
4) Place the shrimps on the double layer rack and cook for 8 minutes.
5) Serve with mayonnaise (optional).

Nutrition information:

- Calories per serving: 148
- Carbs: 9.8g

- Protein: 21.9g
- Fat: 2.3g

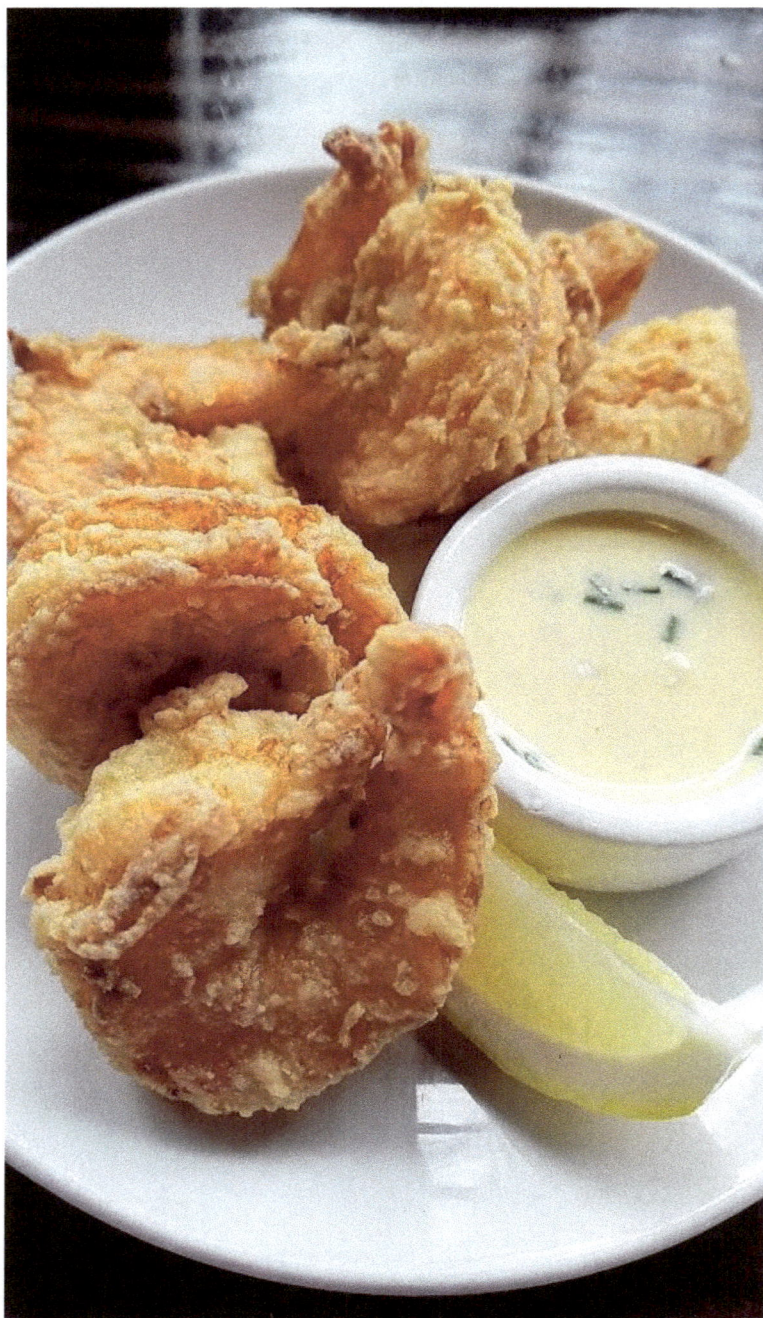

Pesto Basted Shrimp about the Grill

Servings per Recipe: 4

Cooking Time: 16 minutes

Ingredients:

- 1 cup pesto /130G
- 1/4 cup chopped fresh basil /32.5G
- 1-lb extra-large shrimp, peeled and deveined /450G
- bamboo skewers, soaked in water
- Extra-virgin extra virgin olive oil, for drizzling
- Freshly ground black pepper

Instructions:

1) Thread shrimp into skewers and set on skewer rack. Shower with oil, season with pepper and salt to taste.
2) At 360° F or 183°C cook for 8 minutes. Turnover halfway through cooking time while sprinkling the shrimps with pesto.
3) Dress with fresh basil, serve and enjoy.

Nutrition Information:

- Calories per Serving: 544
- Carbs: 9.6g
- Protein: 7.0g
- Fat: 53.0

Pesto Sauce Over Fish Filet

Serves: 3

Cooking Time: 20 minutes

Ingredients:

- 1 bunch of fresh basil
- 1 cup organic olive oil /250ML
- 1 tablespoon parmesan cheese, grated /15G
- 2 cloves of garlic,
- 2 tablespoons pine nuts /30G
- 3 white fish fillets
- Salt and pepper to taste

Instructions:

1) Get a mixing bowl, place all ingredients in it except the fish fillets. Mix properly
2) Beat until smooth.
3) Place the fish in a baking pan and pour in the pesto sauce.
4) Place in the air fryer and cook for 20 minutes at 400° F or 205°C .

Nutrition information:

- Calories per serving: 191
- Carbohydrates: 9.5g
- Protein: 8.2g

- Fat: 13.3g

Pina Colada Sauce Over Coconut Shrimps

Servings per Recipe: 4

Cooking Time: 6 minutes

Ingredients:

- ¼ cup pineapple chunks, drained /32.5G
- ½ cup cornstarch /65G
- ¾ cups panko bread crumbs /88G
- 1 ½ pounds jumbo shrimps, peeled and deveined /675G
- 1 cup shredded coconut flakes /130G
- 1/3 cup light coconut milk /83ML
- 1/3 cup non-fat Greek yogurt /43G
- 2 tablespoons honey /30ML
- 2/3 cup coconut milk /166ML
- Salt and pepper to taste
- Toasted coconut meat for garnish

Instructions:

1) Preheat air fryer to 390° F or 199°C .
2) In a large Ziploc bag, place the shrimps and cornstarch, shake excellently.
3) In a mixing bowl, add coconut milk and honey. Stir well to combine. Set aside.

4) In another mixing bowl, mix the coconut flakes and bread crumbs. Set aside.

5) Dip the shrimps inside the milk mixture then dip inside the bread crumbs. Coat properly.

6) Place inside the double layer rack and cook for 6 minutes.

7) Meanwhile, combine other ingredients to make the dipping sauce.

Nutrition information:

- Calories per serving: 493
- Carbs: 21.4g
- Protein: 38.9g
- Fat: 27.9g

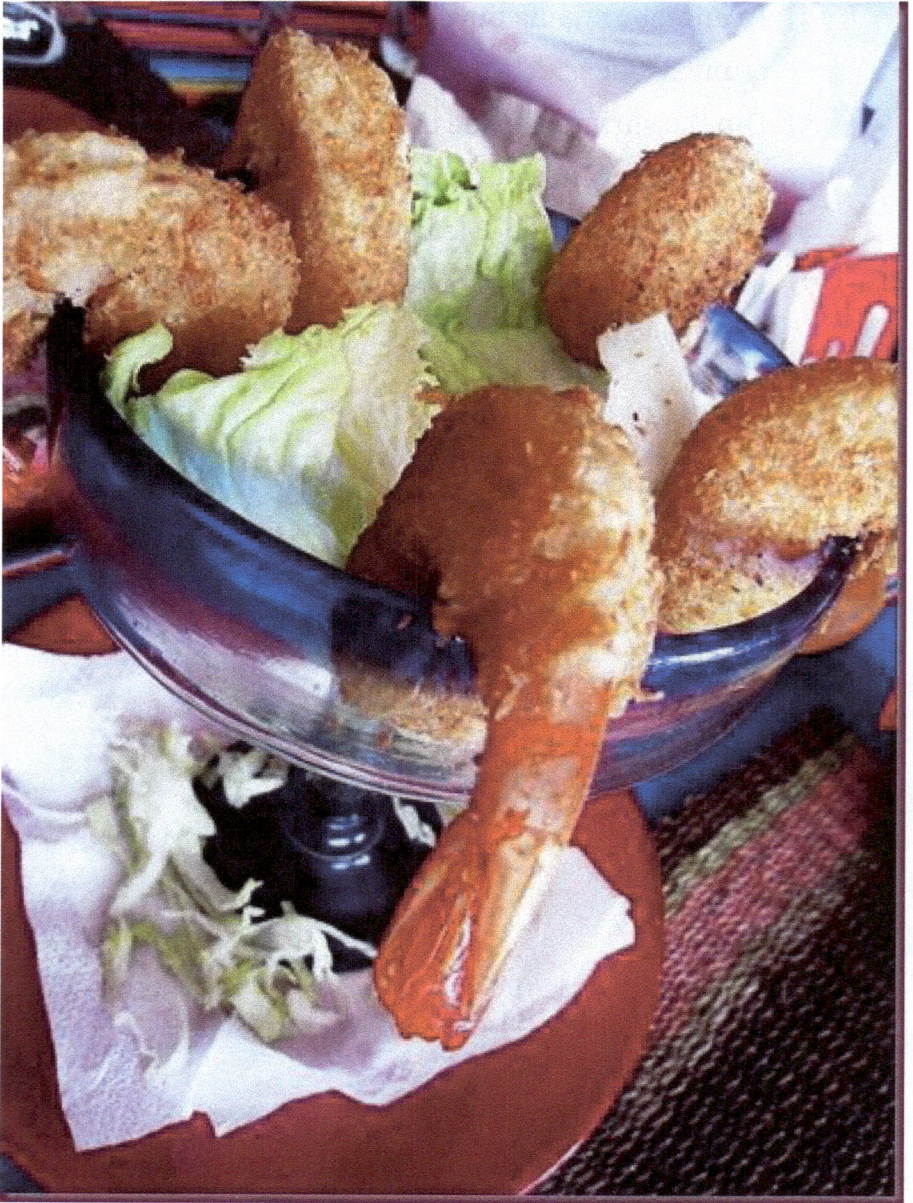

Quick 'n Easy Tuna-Mac Casserole

Servings per Recipe: 4

Cooking Time: 20 minutes

Ingredients:

- 1/2 (10.75 ounces or 322.5 ML) can condensed cream of chicken soup
- 1-1/2 cups cooked macaroni /195G
- 1/2 (5 ounces or 150G) can tuna, drained
- 1/2 cup shredded Cheddar cheese /65G
- 3/4 cup French fried onions /98G

Instructions:

1) Lightly grease the baking pan with oil.
2) Mix soup, tuna, and macaroni in a pan. Sprinkle cheese on top.
3) At 360° F or 183°C cook for 15 minutes. Bring out.
4) Sprinkle fried onions.
5) Cook for an additional 5 minutes.
6) Serve and enjoy.

Nutrition Information:

- Calories per Serving: 411
- Carbs: 37.1g
- Protein: 11.5g

- Fat: 28.5g

Salad Nicosia With Peppery Halibut

Servings per Recipe: 6

Cooking Time: 15

Ingredients:

- 1 ½ pounds halibut fillets /675G
- 1 cup cherry tomatoes, halved /130G
- 2 pounds mixed vegetables /900G
- 2 tablespoons extra virgin olive oil /30ML
- 4 cups torn lettuce leaves /520G
- 4 large hard-boiled eggs, peeled and sliced
- Salt and pepper to taste

Instructions:

1) Preheat mid-air fryer to 390 ° F or 199°C .
2) Place the grill pan in the air fryer.
3) Sprinkle the halibut with salt and pepper. Brush with oil.
4) Place on the grill.
5) Envelop the fish fillet with the mixed vegetables and cook for 15 minutes.
6) Prepare the salad by serving the fish fillet with grilled mixed vegetables, lettuce, cherry tomatoes, and hard-boiled eggs.

Nutrition information:

- Calories per serving: 312
- Carbs:16.8 g
- Protein: 19.8g
- Fat: 18.3g

Crispy Asparagus Dipped in Paprika-Garlic Spice

Serves: 5

Cooking Time: 15 minutes

Ingredients:

- ¼ cup almond flour /32.5G
- ½ teaspoon garlic powder /2.5G
- ½ teaspoon smoked paprika /2.5G
- 10 medium asparagus, trimmed
- 2 large eggs, beaten
- 2 tablespoons parsley, chopped /30G
- Salt and pepper to taste

Instructions:

1) Preheat the air fryer for 5 minutes.
2) Add the parsley, garlic powder, almond flour, and smoked paprika to a bowl and mix properly. Season with salt and pepper.
3) Dip the asparagus in the whisked eggs and turnover in the almond flour mixture to coat evenly.
4) Place in air fryer basket.
5) Cook for 15 at 350° F or 177°C .

Nutrition information:

- Calories per serving: 114
- Carbohydrates: 4.9g
- Protein: 5.2g
- Fat: 8.2g

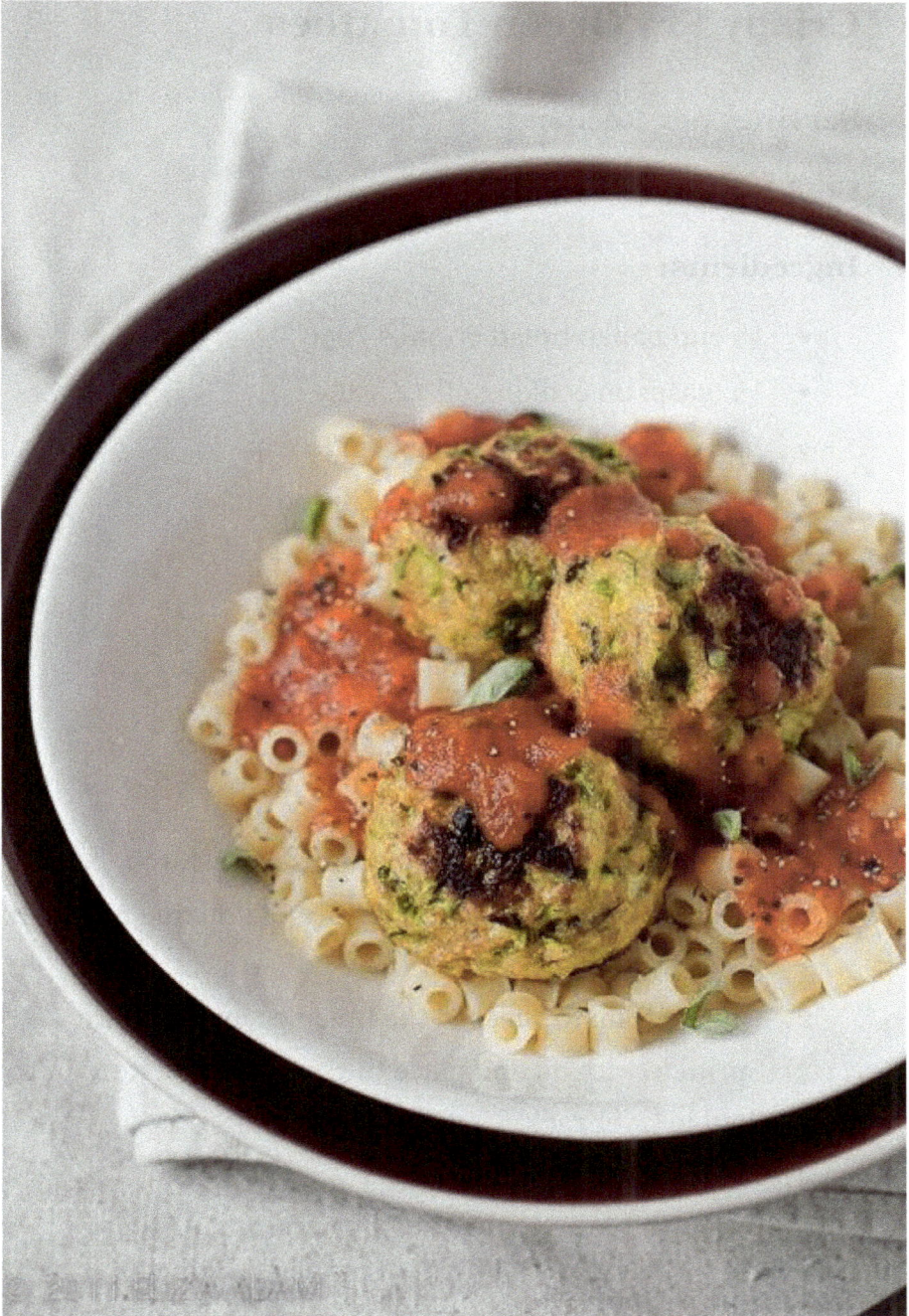

Crispy Fry Green Tomatoes

Servings per Recipe: 1

Cooking Time: 7 minutes

Ingredients:

- ½ cup panko bread crumbs /65G
- ½ teaspoon cooking oil /2.5ML
- ½ teaspoon dried basil, ground /2.5G
- ½ teaspoon dried oregano, ground /2.5G
- ½ teaspoon granulated onion /2.5G
- 1 medium-sized green tomato, sliced
- 3 tablespoons cornstarch /45G
- Salt and pepper to taste

Instructions:

1) Combine the panko bread crumbs, cornstarch, basil, oregano, onion, salt and pepper in na mixing bowl. Mix properly.
2) Dip the tomato slices in the bread crumb mixture.
3) Sprinkle with oil and place the dredged tomatoes in the double layer rack.
4) Place in the air fryer.
5) Cook for 7 minutes at 330° F or 166°C .

Nutrition information:

- Calories per serving: 260
- Carbs: 54.1g
- Protein: 5.4g
- Fat: 3.4g

Crispy Onion Seasoned with Paprika 'n Cajun

Serves: 4

Cooking Time: 20 Minutes

Ingredients:

- ¼ cup coconut milk /62.5ML
- ½ teaspoon Cajun seasoning /2.5G
- ¾ cup almond flour /88G
- 1 ½ teaspoon paprika /7.5G
- 1 large white onion
- 1 teaspoon garlic powder /5G
- 2 large eggs, beaten
- Salt and pepper to taste

Instructions:

1) Peel the onion
2) Add the coconut milk and the eggs to a mixing bowl and whisk well.
3) Soak the onion inside the egg mixture.
4) In another bowl, combine the almond flour, paprika garlic powder, Cajun seasoning, salt and pepper.
5) Dredge the onion in the almond flour mixture.
6) Grease with cooking spray.
7) Place in mid-air fryer.

8) Cook for 20 Minutes at 350° F or 177°C .

Nutrition information:

- Calories per serving: 93
- Carbohydrates: 6.7g
- Protein: 2.6g
- Fat: 6.2g

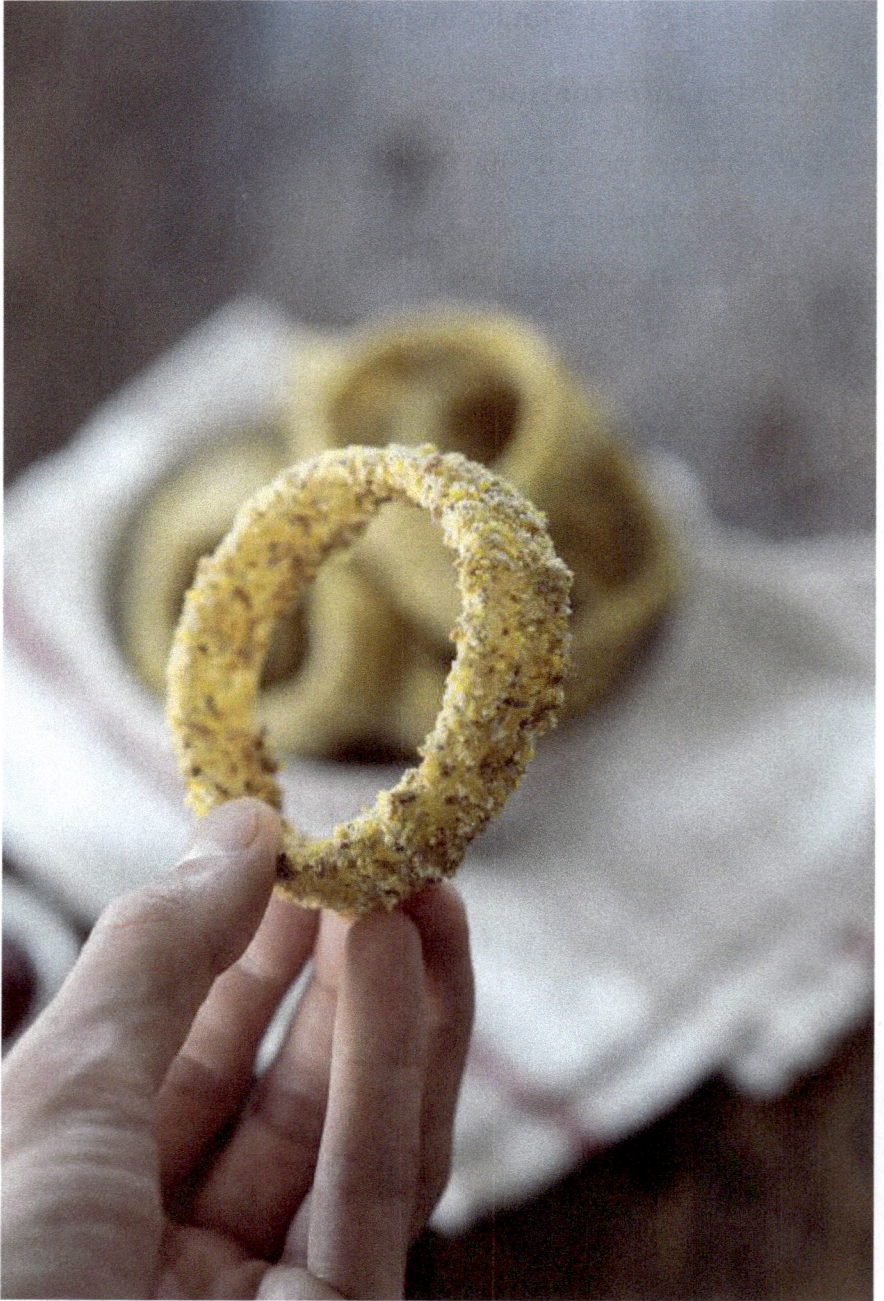

Crispy Vegetarian Ravioli

Serves: 4

Cooking Time: 6 minutes

Ingredients:

- ¼ cup aquafaba /62.5ML
- ½ cup panko bread crumbs /65G
- 1 teaspoon dried basil /5G
- 1 teaspoon dried oregano /5G
- 1 teaspoon garlic powder /5G
- 2 teaspoons nutritional yeast /10G
- 8-ounces vegan ravioli /240G
- cooking spray
- salt and pepper to taste

Instructions:

1) Lay aluminium foil within the air fryer basket and spray with oil.
2) Preheat the air fryer to 400° F or 205°C .
3) Add the panko bread crumbs, nutritional yeast, basil, oregano, and garlic powder to a bowl and mix properly. Season with salt and pepper to taste.
4) Squeeze the aquafaba in a bowl
5) Lightly cover the ravioli with the aquafaba and then turn over in the panko mixture.

6) Spray with oil and place in the air fryer.

7) Cook for 6 minutes ensuring you shake the mid-air fryer basket halfway through cooking time.

Nutrition information:

- Calories per serving: 82
- Carbohydrates: 12.18g
- Protein:3.36 g
- Fat: 2.15g

Crispy Veggie Tempura Style

Servings per Recipe: 3

Cooking Time: 15 minutes

Ingredients:

- ¼ teaspoon salt /1.25G
- ¾ cup club soda /188ML
- 1 ½ cups panko bread crumbs /195G
- 1 cup broccoli florets /130G
- 1 egg, beaten
- 1 red bell pepper, cut into strips
- 1 small sweet potato, peeled and cut into thick slices
- 1 small zucchini, cut into thick slices
- 1/3 cup all-purpose flour /43G
- 2/3 cup cornstarch /87G
- Non-stick cooking spray

Instructions:

1) Lightly cover the vegetables with cornstarch and also in the all-purpose flour mixture.
2) Dip each vegetable in the blend of egg and club soda before dredging in bread crumbs.
3) Place the vegetables on the double layer rack and brush with cooking oil.
4) Place inside the air fryer.

5) Close and cook for 20 minutes at 330° F or 166°C .

Nutrition information:

- Calories per serving:277
- Carbs: 51.6g
- Protein: 7.2g
- Fat: 4.2g

Salted Beet Chips

Servings per Recipe: 2

Cooking Time: 6 minutes

Ingredients:

- 1 tablespoon cooking oil /15ML
- 1-pound beets, peeled and sliced /450G
- Salt and pepper to taste

Instructions:

1) Place all ingredients in a bowl and mix everything to coat properly.
2) Place the sliced beets inside double layer rack.
3) Place the rack with all the beets in the air fryer.
4) Close the air fryer and cook for 6 minutes at 390° F or 199°C .

Nutrition information:

- Calories per serving: 167
- Carbs: 23.8g
- Protein: 4.1g
- Fat: 7.2g

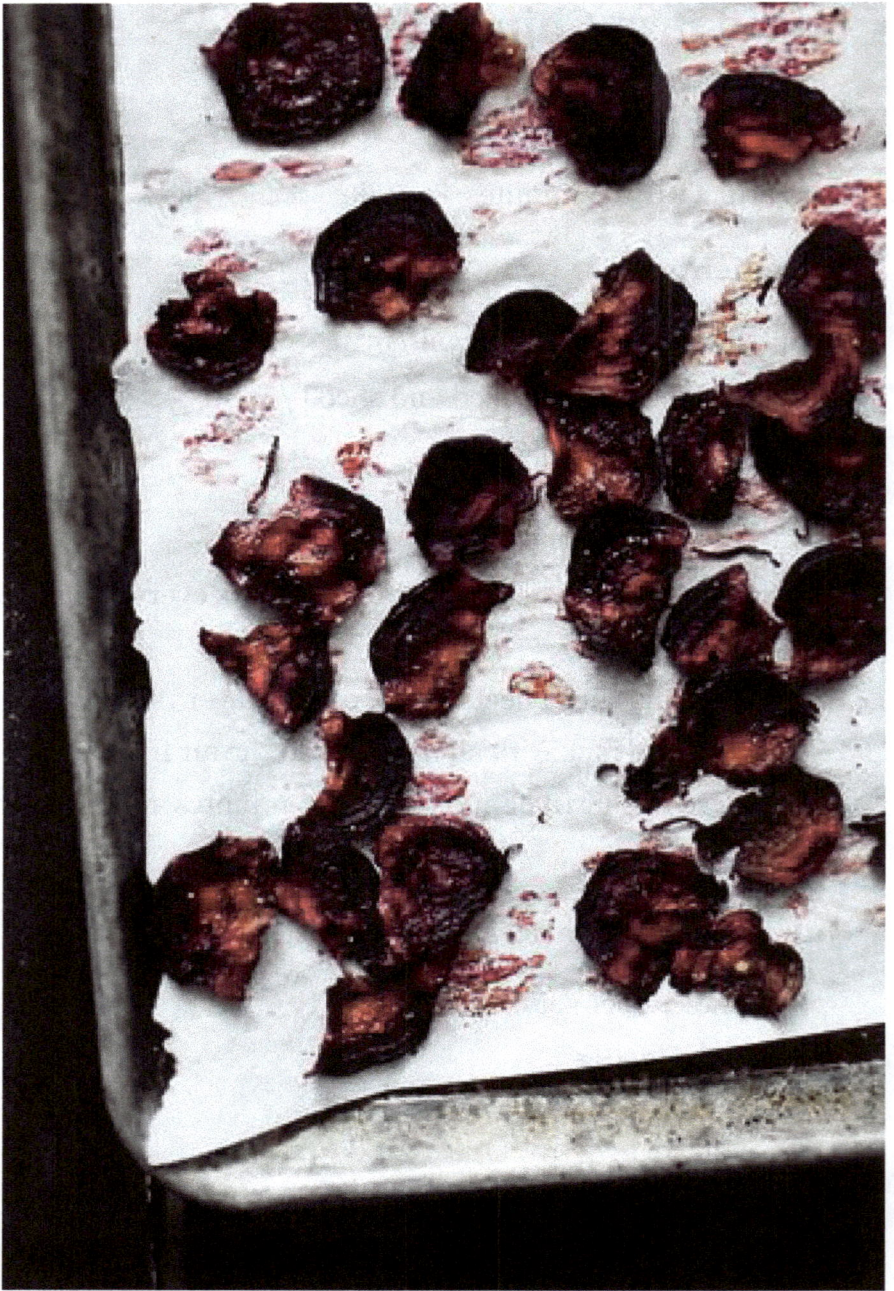

Salted Garlic Zucchini Fries

Serves: 6

Cooking Time: 15

Ingredients:

- ¼ teaspoon garlic powder /1.25G
- ½ cup almond flour /65G
- 2 large egg whites, beaten
- 3 medium zucchinis, sliced into fry sticks
- Salt and pepper to taste

Instructions:

1) Preheat the air fryer for 5 minutes.
2) Mix all ingredients in a bowl until the zucchini fries are well coated.
3) Place in the air fryer basket.
4) Cook at 425° F or 219°C for 15 minutes.

Nutrition information:

- Calories per serving:11
- Carbohydrates: 1g
- Protein: 0.1g
- Fat: 1.5g

Salted Potato-Kale Nuggets

Serves: 4

Cooking Time: 20 minutes

Ingredients:

- ¼ teaspoon salt /1.25G
- 1 clove of garlic, minced
- 1 teaspoon extra-virgin organic olive oil /5ML
- 1/8 cup almond milk /31.25ML
- 1/8 teaspoon black pepper /0.625G
- 2 cups boiled potatoes, finely chopped /260G
- 4 cups kale, rinsed and chopped /520G
- cooking spray

Instructions:

1) Preheat the air fryer to 400° F or 205°C .
2) Place an aluminium foil at the base of the air fryer basket and make holes in the foil to allow air circulation.
3) Place a pan over heat, add oil, sauté the garlic for two main minutes, add the kale until it withers. Transfer into a large bowl.
4) Add the potatoes and almond milk. Season with salt and pepper to taste.
5) Form balls with the constituents and spray with olive oil.

6) Place inside air fryer and cook for 20 minutes or until golden brown.

Nutrition information:

- Calories per serving: 88
- Carbohydrates: 18.05g
- Protein:2.13 g
- Fat: 0.81g

Savory Zucchini-Bell Pepper Medley

Serves: 4

Cooking Time: 15

Ingredients:

- 1 green pepper, seeded and julienned
- 1 large zucchini
- 1 red pepper, seeded and julienned
- 1 teaspoon mixed herbs /5G
- 1 teaspoon prepared mustard /5G
- 2 teaspoons minced garlic /10G
- 6 tablespoons organic olive oil /90ML
- Salt and pepper to taste

Instructions:

1) Preheat the air fryer for 5 minutes.
2) Place all ingredients in a baking pan and mix to combine.
3) Place the baking pan in the air fryer.
4) Cook at 350°F or 177°C for 15 minutes.

Nutrition information:

- Calories per serving: 218
- Carbohydrates: 6.2g
- Protein: 1.7g
- Fat: 20.7g

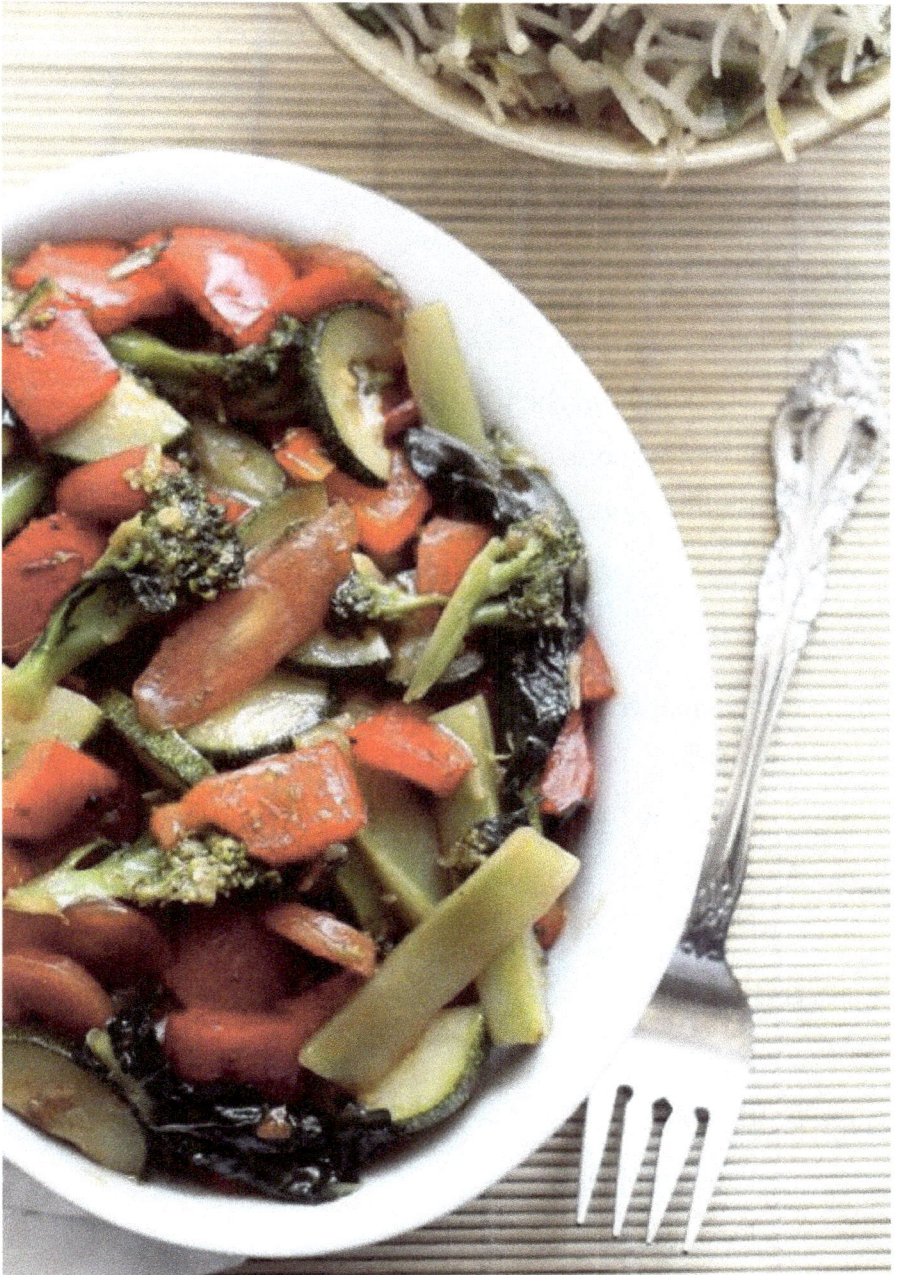

Scrumptiously Healthy Chips

Serves: 2

Cooking Time: 10

Ingredients

- 1 bunch of kale
- 1 teaspoon garlic powder /5G
- 2 tablespoons almond flour /30G
- 2 tablespoons extra virgin olive oil /30ML
- Salt and pepper to taste

Instructions:

1) Preheat the air fryer for 5 minutes.
1) 2 Grab a bowl and combine all ingredients. Mix well to combine making sure the kale leaves are well coated.
2) Place in the fryer basket and cook for 10 minutes until crispy.

Nutrition information:

- Calories per serving: 183
- Carbohydrates: 3.1g
- Protein: 4.5g
- Fat: 16.9g

Capers 'n Olives Topped Flank Steak

Servings per Recipe: 4

Cooking Time: 45 minutes

Ingredients:

- 1 anchovy fillet, minced
- 1 clove of garlic, minced
- 1 cup pitted olives /250G
- 1 tablespoon capers, minced /15G
- 1/3 cup extra virgin olive oil /83ML
- 2 pounds flank steak, pounded /900G
- 2 tablespoons fresh oregano /30G
- 2 tablespoons garlic powder /30G
- 2 tablespoons onion powder /30G
- 2 tablespoons smoked paprika /30G
- Salt and pepper to taste

Instructions:

1) Preheat air fryer to 390° F or 199°C .
2) Place the grill pan in the mid-air fryer.
3) Season the steak with salt and pepper. Rub the oregano, paprika, onion powder, and garlic powder lavishly on the steak.

4) Place in the grill pan and cook for 45 minutes. Turnover the meat every 10 minutes to ensure even cooking.

5) Mix the olive oil, olives, capers, garlic, and anchovy fillets.

6) Serve the steak and dress using tapenade.

Nutrition information:

- Calories per serving: 553
- Carbs: 11.6g
- Protein: 51.5g
- Fat: 33.4g

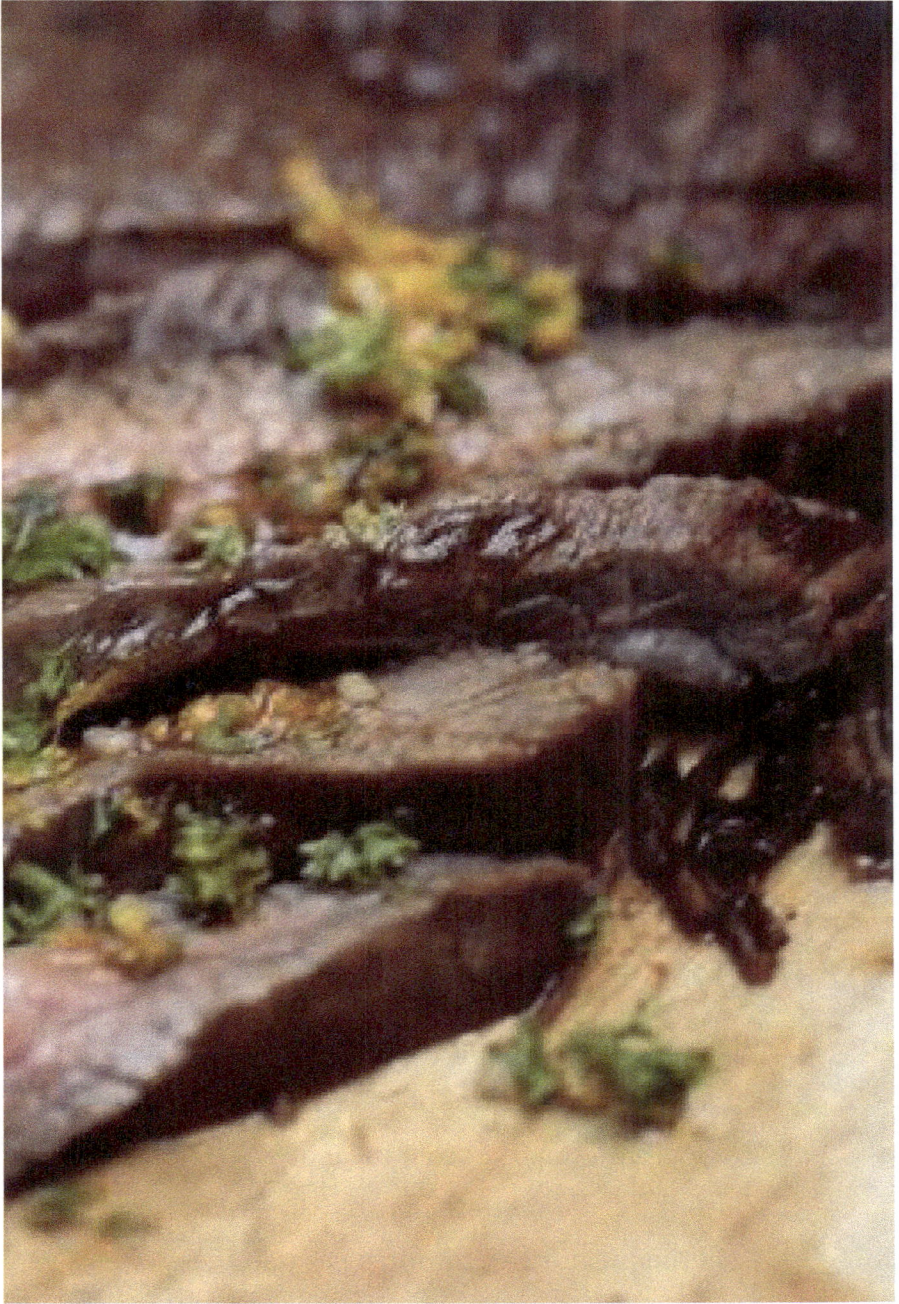

Caraway, Sichuan 'n Cumin Lamb Kebabs

Servings per Recipe: 3

Cooking Time: 1 hour

Ingredients:

1 ½ pounds lamb shoulder, bones removed and cut into pieces /675G

1 tablespoon Sichuan peppercorns /15G

1 teaspoon sugar /5G

2 tablespoons cumin seeds, toasted /30G

2 teaspoons caraway seeds, toasted /10G

2 teaspoons crushed red pepper flakes /10G

Salt and pepper to taste

Instructions:

1) Place all ingredients in a bowl, add the meat and place in the fridge to marinate for a couple of hours.
2) Preheat mid-air fryer to 390° F or 199°C .
3) Place the grill pan in the air fryer.
4) Grill the meat for 15 minutes per batch.
5) Flip the meat every 8 minutes for even grilling.

Nutrition information:

- Calories per serving: 465
- Carbs:7.7g
- Protein: 22.8g
- Fat: 46.9g

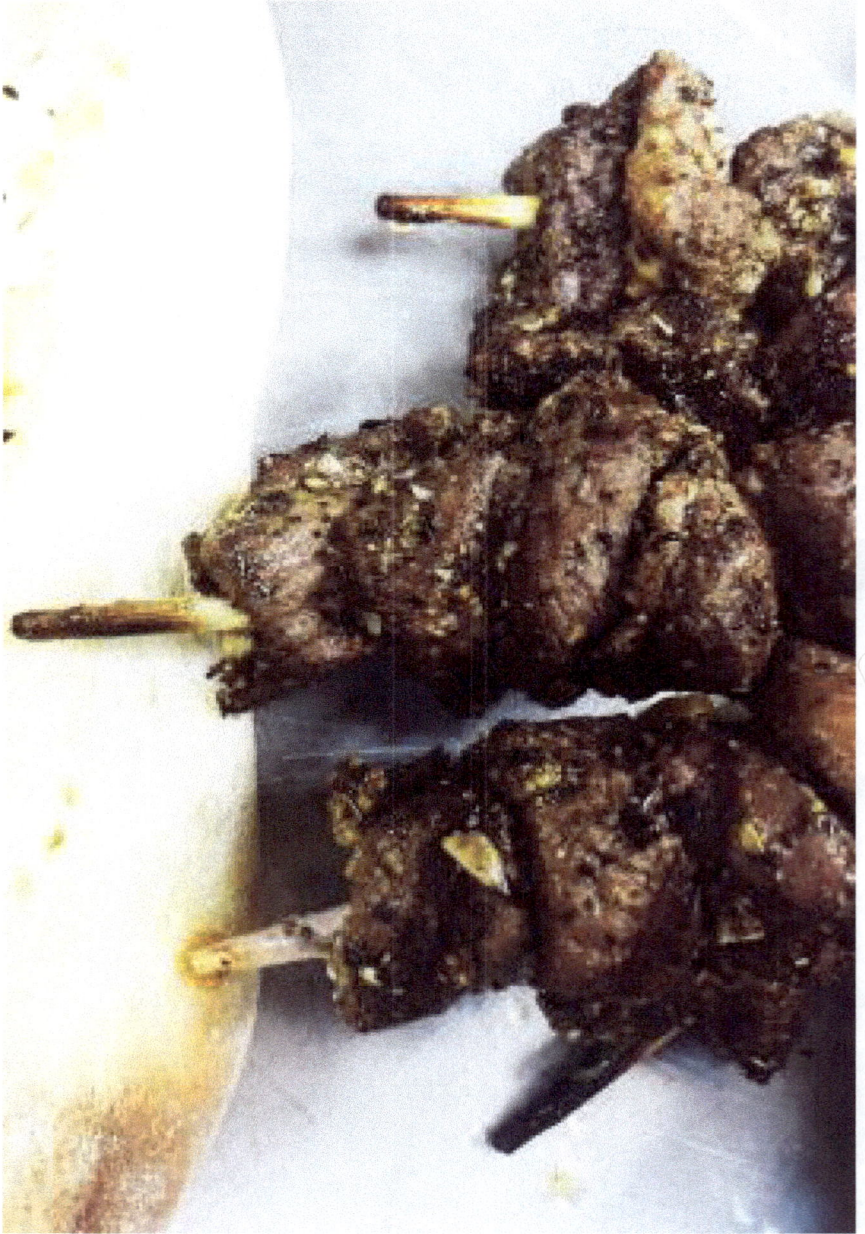

Champagne-Vinegar Marinated Skirt Steak

Servings per Recipe: 2

Cooking Time: 40 minutes

Ingredients:

- ¼ cup Dijon mustard /32.5G
- 1 tablespoon rosemary leaves /15G
- 1-pound skirt steak, trimmed /450G
- 2 tablespoons champagne vinegar /30ML
- Salt and pepper to taste

Instructions:

1) Place all ingredients in a Ziploc bag and marinate in the fridge for a couple of hours.
2) Preheat air fryer to 390° F or 199°C .
3) Place the grill pan in the mid-air fryer.
4) Grill the skirt steak for 20 minutes per batch.
5) Flip the beef halfway through the cooking time.

Nutrition information:

- Calories per serving: 516
- Carbs: 4.2g
- Protein: 60.9g
- Fat: 28.4g

Char-Grilled Skirt Steak with Fresh Herbs

Servings per Recipe: 3

Cooking Time: 30 Minutes

Ingredients:

- 1 ½ pounds skirt steak, trimmed /675G
- 1 tablespoon lemon zest /15G
- 1 tablespoon olive oil /15G
- 2 cups fresh herbs like tarragon, sage, and mint, chopped /260G
- 4 cloves of garlic, minced
- Salt and pepper to taste

Instructions:

1) Preheat mid-air fryer to 390° F or 199°C .
2) Place the grill pan in the air fryer.
3) Season the steak with salt, pepper, lemon zest, herbs, and garlic.
4) Brush with oil.
5) Grill for 15 minutes and if needed cook in batches.

Nutrition information:

- Calories per serving: 478
- Carbs: 18g

- Protein: 25g
- Fat: 34g

Charred Onions 'n Steak Cube BBQ

Servings per Recipe: 3

Cooking Time: 40 minutes

Ingredients:

- 1 cup red onions, cut into wedges /130G
- 1 tablespoon dry mustard /15G
- 1 tablespoon organic olive oil /15ML
- 1-pound boneless beef sirloin, cut into cubes /450G
- Salt and pepper to taste

Instructions:

1) Preheat air fryer to 390° F or 199°C .
2) Place the grill pan in the air fryer.
3) Add all ingredients to the bowl and mix properly.
4) Place on the grill pan and cook for 40 minutes.
5) Shake halfway through the cooking time for even brownness.

Nutrition information:

- Calories per serving: 260
- Carbs: 5.2g
- Protein: 35.7g
- Fat: 10.7g

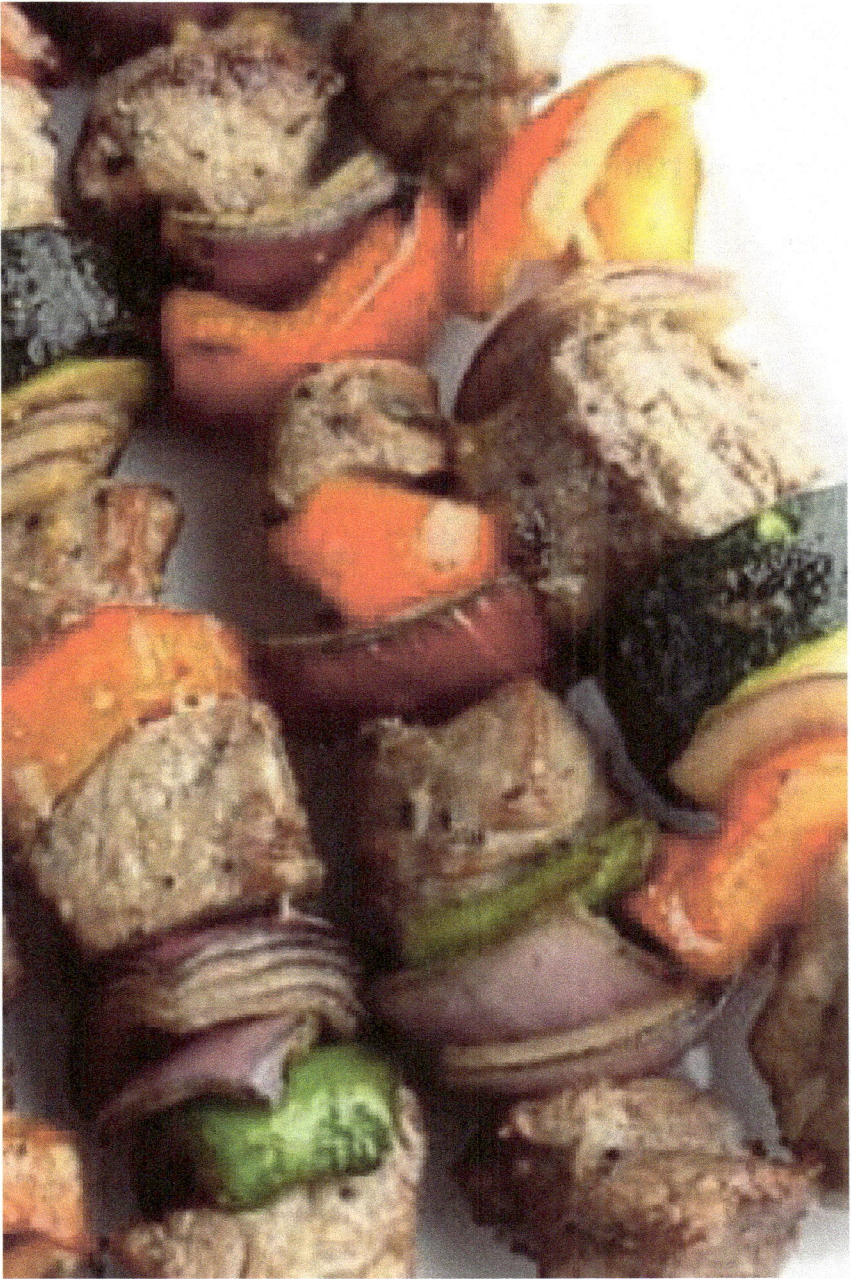

Maple 'n Soy Marinated Beef

Servings per Recipe: 4

Cooking Time: 45 minutes

Ingredients:

- 2 pounds sirloin flap steaks, pounded /900G
- 3 tablespoons balsamic vinegar /45ML
- 3 tablespoons maple syrup /45ML
- 3 tablespoons soy sauce /45ML
- 4 cloves of garlic, minced

Instructions:

1) Preheat mid-air fryer to 390° F or 199°C .
2) Place the grill pan in the air fryer.
3) Place the flap steaks in a deep pan and season with soy sauce, balsamic vinegar, and maple syrup, and garlic.
4) Place the grill pan in the air fryer and cook for 15 minutes in batches.

Nutrition information:

- Calories per serving: 331
- Carbs: 9g
- Protein: 31g
- Fat: 19g

Maras Pepper Lamb Kebab Recipe from Turkey

Servings per Recipe: 2

Cooking Time: 15

Ingredients:

- 1-lb lamb meat, cut into 2-inch cubes /450G
- Kosher salt
- Freshly cracked black pepper
- 2 tablespoons Maras pepper, or 2 teaspoons other dried chili powder combined with 1 tablespoon paprika /30G OR 10G+15G
- 1 teaspoon minced garlic /5G
- 2 tablespoons roughly chopped fresh mint /30G
- 1/2 cup extra-virgin essential olive oil, divided /125ML
- 1/2 cup dried apricots, cut into medium dice /65G

Instructions:

1) Add pepper, salt, and 50% of organic olive oil in a bowl. Add lamb and mix well to coat. Thread lamb into 4 skewers.

2) Cook for 5 minutes at 390°F or 199°C to the desired doneness.

3) All mix the remaining oil, mint, garlic, Maras pepper, and apricots in a bowl. Mix well. Add cooked lamb. Season with salt and pepper. Mix well again.

4) Serve and enjoy.

Nutrition Information:

- Calories per Serving: 602
- Carbs: 25.8g
- Protein: 40.3g
- Fat: 37.5g

Meat Balls with Mint Yogurt Dip From Morocco

Servings per Recipe: 2

Cooking Time: 25 minutes

Ingredients:

- ¼ cup bread crumbs /32.5G
- ¼ cup sour cream /62.5ML
- ½ cup Greek yogurt /125ML
- 1 clove of garlic, minced
- 1 egg, beaten
- 1 tablespoon mint, chopped /15G
- 1 teaspoon cayenne /5G
- 1 teaspoon ground coriander /5G
- 1 teaspoon ground cumin /5G
- 1 teaspoon red chili paste /5G
- 1-pound ground beef /450G
- 2 cloves of garlic, minced
- 2 tablespoons flat-leaf parsley, chopped /30G
- 2 tablespoons buttermilk /30ML
- 2 tablespoons honey /30ML
- 2 tablespoons mint
- Salt and pepper to taste

Instructions:

1) Add the ground beef, cumin, coriander, cayenne, red chili paste, minced garlic, parsley, chopped mint, egg, and bread crumbs in a bowl. Season with salt and pepper to taste. Form small balls with your hands. Place in a fridge for about 30 minutes.

2) Preheat the air fryer to 330° F or 166°C .

3) Place the meatballs in a mid-air fryer basket and cook for 25 minutes. Shake the air fryer frequently to allow roasting evenly

4) Now, mix the Greek yogurt, sour cream, buttermilk, mint, garlic, and honey in a very bowl. Season with salt and pepper.

5) Serve the meatballs with the yogurt sauce.

Nutrition information:

- Calories per serving: 779
- Carbs: 28.5g
- Protein: 65g
- Fat: 45g

Meatballs 'n Parmesan-Cheddar Pizza

Servings per Recipe: 4

Cooking Time: 15 minutes

Ingredients:

- 1 prebaked 6-inch pizza crust
- 1 teaspoon garlic powder /5G
- 1 teaspoon Italian seasoning /5G
- 4 tbsp grated Parmesan cheese /60G
- 1 small onion, halved and sliced
- 1/2 can (8 ounces) pizza sauce /240G
- 6 frozen fully cooked Italian meatballs (1/2 ounce each), thawed and halved /15G EACH
- 1/2 cup shredded part-skim mozzarella cheese /65G
- 1/2 cup shredded cheddar cheese /65G

Instructions:

1) Grease the baking pan of the air fryer lightly with cooking spray.
2) Spread pizza crust evenly on the pan. Spread sauce on it. Sprinkle with parmesan, Italian seasoning, and garlic powder.
3) Add meatballs and onion to the top. Sprinkle the remaining cheese.

4) For 15 minutes, cook on preheated 390 ° F or 199°C air fryer.

5) Serve and enjoy

Nutrition Information:

- Calories per Serving: 324
- Carbs: 28.0g
- Protein: 17.0g
- Fat: 16.0g

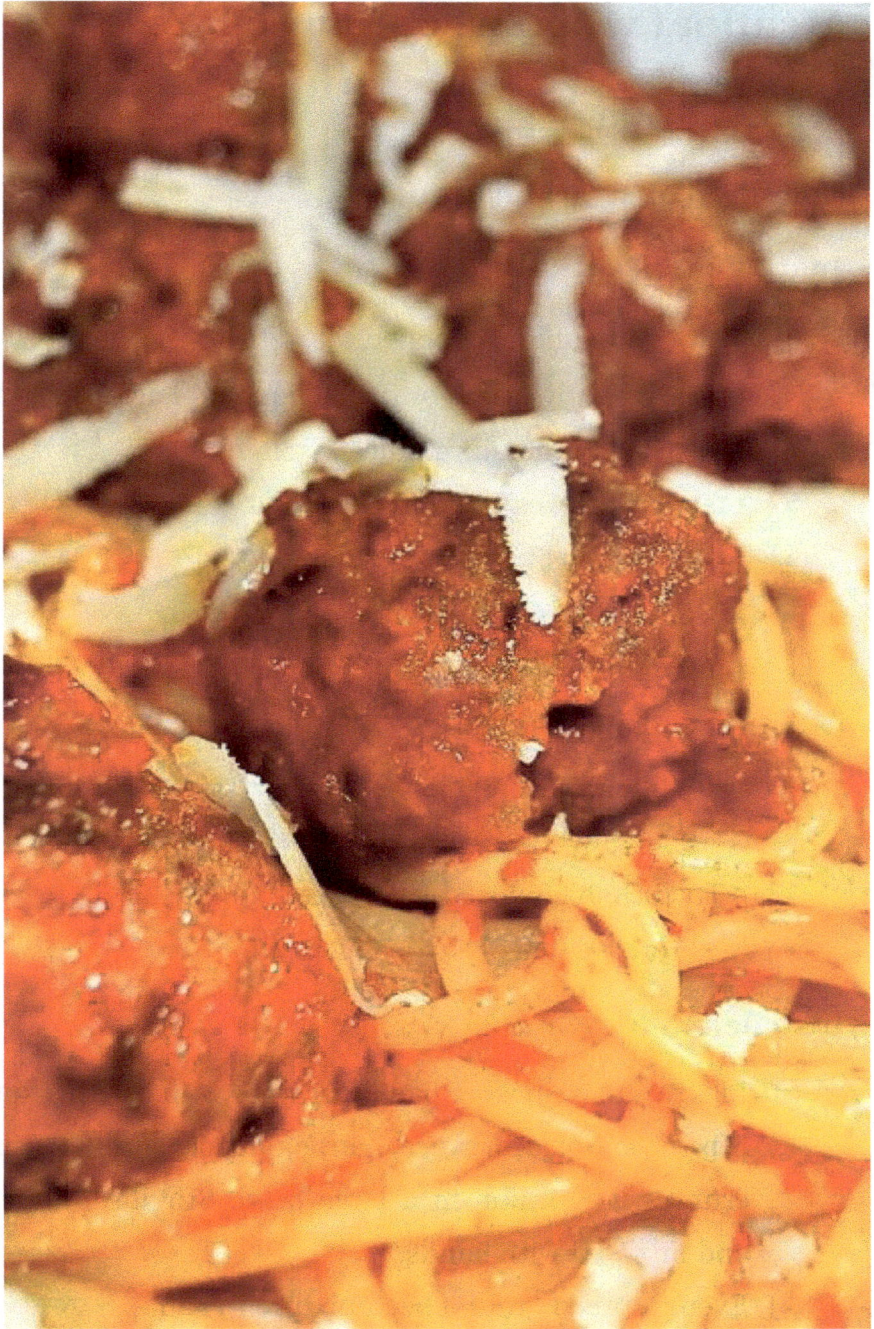

Meatloaf with Sweet-Sour Glaze

Servings per Recipe: 3

Cooking Time: 30 Minutes

Ingredients:

- ½ medium onion, chopped
- ½ Tbsp lightly dried (or fresh chopped) Parsley /7.5G
- 1 Tbsp Worcestershire sauce /15ML
- 1 tsp (or 2 cloves) minced garlic /5G
- 1 tsp dried basil /5G
- 1/3 cup Kellogg's corn flakes crumbs /43G
- 1-2 tsp freshly ground black pepper /2.5G
- 1-2 tsp salt /2.5G
- 1-pound lean ground beef (93% fat-free), raw /450G
- 3 tsp Splenda (or Truvia) brown sugar blend /15G
- 5 Tbsp Heinz reduced-sugar ketchup /75ML
- 8-oz tomato sauce, divided /240ML

Instructions:

1) Lightly grease baking pan of air fryer with cooking spray.
2) Mix 6-oz tomato sauce, garlic, pepper, salt, cornflake crumbs, and onion in a large bowl. Stir in ground beef and mix well with hands.
3) Evenly spread ground beef mixture in pan

4) Place all ingredients in a medium-sized bowl, mix to produce a glaze. Pour the ground beef.

5) Cover the pan with foil.

6) Cook for 15 minutes at 360° F or 183°C . Remove foil and continue cooking for another 10 minutes.

7) Let it cool for 5 minutes.

8) Serve and enjoy

Nutrition Information:

- Calories per Serving: 427
- Carbs: 25.7g
- Protein: 42.5g
- Fat: 17.1

Smoked Brisket with Dill Pickles

Servings per Recipe: 6

Cooking Time: one hour

Ingredients:

- ¼ teaspoon liquid smoke /1.25ML
- 1 cup dill pickles /130G
- 3 pounds flat-cut brisket /1350G
- Salt and pepper to taste

Instructions:

1) Preheat the air fryer to 390° F or 199°C .
2) Place the grill pan accessory in the mid-air fryer.
3) Season the brisket with liquid smoke, salt, and pepper.
4) Place in the grill pan and cook for 30 minutes per batch.
5) Flip the meat halfway through cooking time for even grilling.
6) Serve with dill pickles.

Nutrition information:

- Calories per serving: 309
- Carbs: 1.2g
- Protein: 49g
- Fat:12 g

Smoked Sausage 'n Shrimp Jambalaya

Servings per Recipe: 4

Cooking Time: 40 minutes

Ingredients:

- salt to taste
- 1 cup chicken broth /250ML
- 1/2 pound peeled and deveined medium shrimp (30-40 per pound) /225G
- 1-1/2 teaspoons organic olive oil /7.5ML
- 1/2 large onion, chopped
- 1/2 cup chopped green bell pepper /65G
- 1/2 cup chopped celery /65G
- 1/2 cup uncooked white rice /65G
- 1-1/2 teaspoons minced garlic /7.5G
- 1-1/2 bay leaves
- 1/4-pound smoked sausage (including Conecuh©), cut into 1/4-inch thick slices /112.5G
- 1/4 teaspoon Cajun seasoning, or to taste /1.25g
- 1/8 teaspoon dried thyme leaves /0.625G
- 1/2 (14.5 ounces) can diced tomatoes with juice /435G

Instructions:

1) Lightly oil baking pan of air fryer with extra virgin olive oil. Add sausage and then for 5 minutes, cook at 360° F or 183°C . Add Cajun seasoning, salt, celery, bell pepper, and onion. Mix well. Cook for another 5 minutes.

2) Add the rice and mix well. Add thyme leaves, bay leaves, chicken broth, garlic, vegetable mixture, and tomatoes with juice while stirring. Cover with foil.

3) Cook for the next 15 minutes.

4) Remove foil, stir in shrimp. Cook for 8 minutes.

5) Let it sit for 5 minutes.

6) Serve, eat and enjoy.

Nutrition Information:

- Calories per Serving: 276
- Carbs: 24.6g
- Protein: 18.4g
- Fat: 11.5g

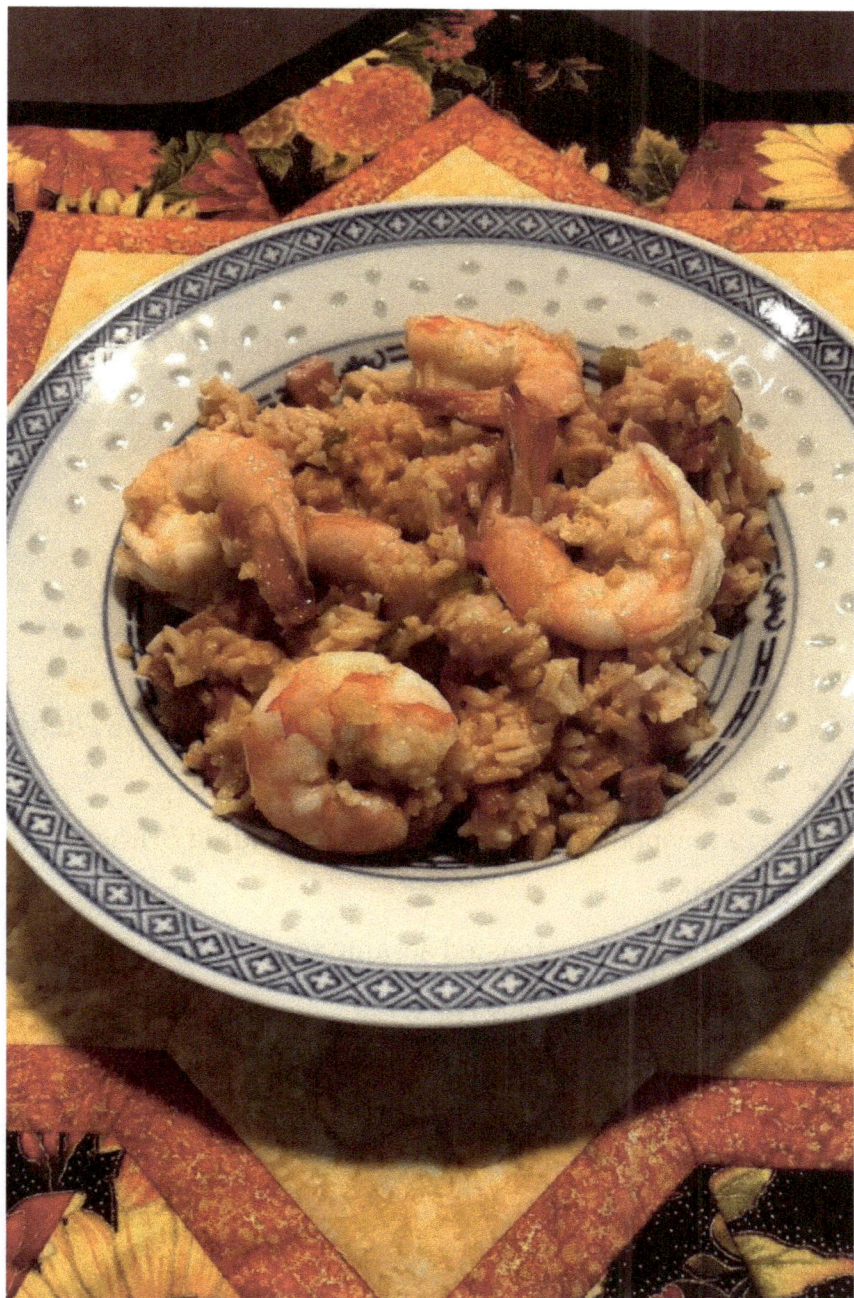

Sriracha-Hoisin Glazed Grilled Beef

Servings per Recipe: 5

Cooking Time: 16 minutes

Ingredients:

- 1-pound flank steak, sliced with an angle 1" x ¼" thick /450G
- 1 tablespoon lime juice /15ML
- 1 chopped green onions
- 1-1/2 teaspoons honey /7.5G
- 1/2 clove garlic, minced
- 1/2 teaspoon kosher salt /2.5G
- 1/2 teaspoon peeled and grated fresh cinnamon /2.5G
- 1/2 teaspoon sesame oil (optional) /2.5ML
- 1/2 teaspoon chile-garlic sauce (including Sriracha®) /2.5ML
- 1-1/2 teaspoons toasted sesame seeds /7.5G
- 1/4 cup hoisin sauce /62.5ML
- 1/4 teaspoon crushed red pepper flakes /1.25G
- 1/8 teaspoon ground black pepper /0.625G

Instructions:

1) Mix pepper, red pepper flakes, chile-garlic sauce, sesame oil, ginger, salt, honey, lime juice, and hoisin sauce. Add steak and mix well to coat. Place in the fridge for 3 hours to marinate.

2) Skewer steak. Place on skewer rack in the air fryer.

3) For 8 minutes, cook on 360° F or 183°C . If need be, cook in batches.

4) Serve and dress with a drizzle of green onions and sesame seeds.

Nutrition Information:

- Calories per Serving: 123
- Carbs: 8.3g
- Protein: 11.7g
- Fat: 4.7g

Tasty Beef Pot Pie

Serves: 6

Cooking Time: 30 Minutes

Ingredients:

- 1 cup almond flour /130G
- 1 green bell pepper, julienned
- 1 onion, chopped
- 1 red bell pepper, julienned
- 1 tablespoon butter /130G
- 1 yellow bell pepper, julienned
- 1-pound ground beef /450G
- 2 beaten eggs
- 2 cloves of garlic, minced
- 4 tablespoons coconut oil /60ML
- Salt and pepper to taste

Instructions:

1) Preheat the air fryer for 5 minutes.
2) Mix the first 9 ingredients in a baking pan. Mix well.
3) Mix the almond flour and eggs into a mixing bowl to make a dough.
4) Press the dough in the beef mixture.
5) Place in the air fryer and cook for 30 minutes at 350° F or 177°C .

Nutrition information:

- Calories per serving: 363
- Carbohydrates: 5.3g
- Protein: 21.3g
- Fat: 28.5g

Tasty Stuffed Gyoza

Servings per Recipe: 4

Cooking Time: 20 Minutes

Ingredients:

- ¼ cup chopped onion /32.5G
- ¼ teaspoon ground cumin /1.25G
- ¼ teaspoon paprika /1.25G
- ½ cup chopped tomatoes /65G
- 1 egg, beaten
- 1 tablespoon extra virgin olive oil /15ML
- 1/8 teaspoon ground cinnamon /.625G
- 2 teaspoons chopped garlic /10G
- 3 ounces chopped cremini mushrooms /90G
- 3 ounces lean ground beef /90G
- 6 pitted green olives, chopped
- 8 gyoza wrappers

Instructions

1) pLace pan over medium heat, add oil to the pan, add the beef and stir for 3 minutes. Add the onions and garlic until weak. Stir in the mushrooms, olives, paprika, cumin, cinnamon, and tomatoes.

2) Close the lid and allow it to simmer for 5 minutes. Allow to cool before making the empanada.

3) Place the meat mixture at the center of the gyoza wrapper. Fold the gyoza wrapper and seal the edges by brushing with egg mixture.
4) Preheat the air fryer to 390° F or 199°C .
5) Place the grill pan accessory.
6) Place the prepared empanada on the grill pan accessory.
7) Cook for 10 Minutes.
8) Flip the empanadas halfway through the cooking time.

Nutrition information:

- Calories per serving: 339
- Carbs: 25g
- Protein: 17g
- Fat: 19g

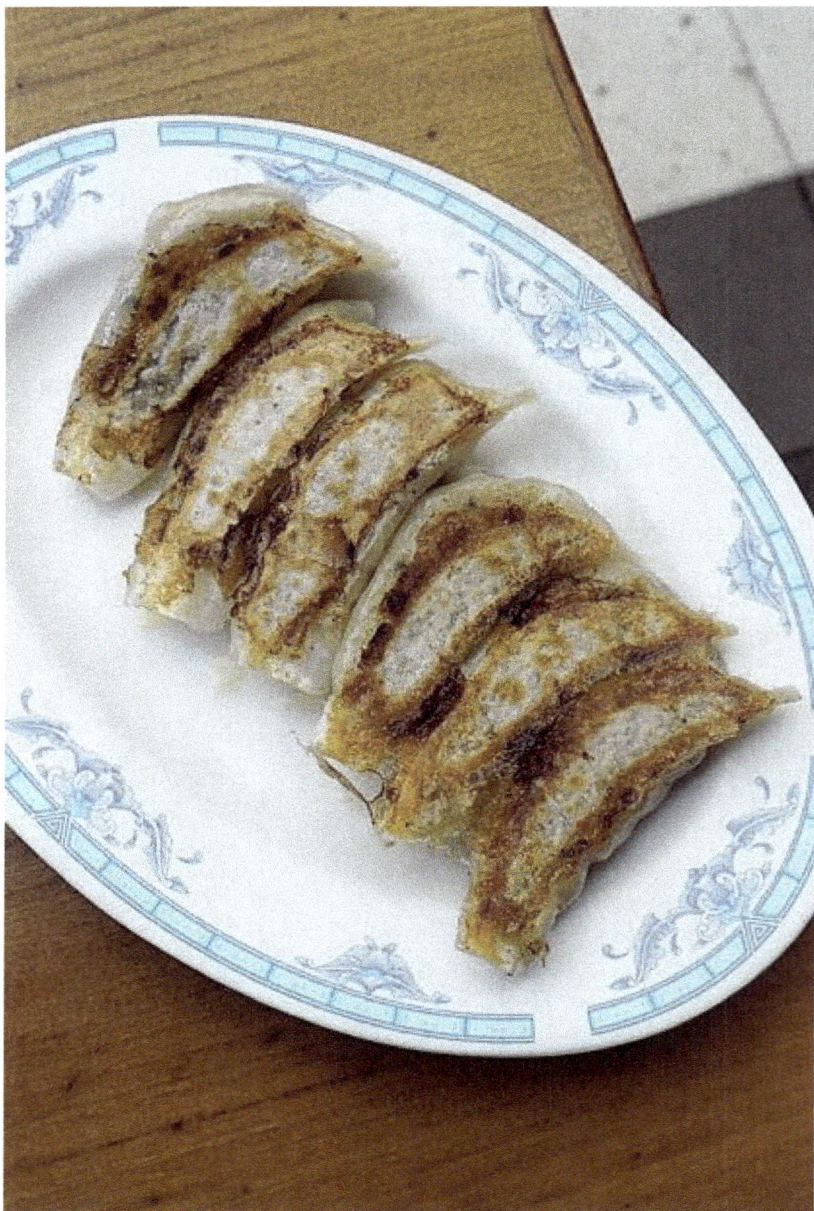

Servings per Recipe: 3

Cooking Time: 25 minutes

Ingredients:

- 1 cup shredded Italian cheese blend /130G
- 1/3 cup milk /83ML
- 1/4 (15 ounces) can crushed tomatoes /450G
- 1/4 (15 ounces) jar Alfredo sauce /450ML
- 1/4 (15 ounces) jar pesto sauce /450ML
- 1-1/2 cups cubed cooked chicken /195G
- 2 tablespoons grated Parmesan cheese /30G
- 2 tablespoons seasoned bread crumbs /30G
- 3/4 cup fresh baby spinach /97
- 3/4 teaspoon organic olive oil /3.75ML
- 4-ounce penne pasta, cooked based on manufacturer's Instructions /120G

Instructions:

1) Add essential olive oil, Parmesan, and bread crumbs to a bowl. Mix well and Set aside.
2) Lightly grease the baking pan of the air fryer. While mixing add milk, pesto sauce, alfredo sauce, tomatoes, spinach, and Italian cheese blend. Mix well. Add in cooked pasta and mix well to coat. Sprinkle bread crumb mixture evenly on top.

3) Cook at 360° F or 183°C for 25 minutes until tops are lightly browned.

4) Serve and enjoy.

Nutrition Information:

- Calories per Serving: 729
- Carbs: 40.7g
- Protein: 45.4g
- Fat: 47.2g

Chicken-Veggie Fusilli Casserole

Servings per Recipe: 3

Cooking Time: 30 Minutes

Ingredients:

- 1 cup frozen mixed vegetables /130G
- 1 tablespoon butter, melted /15ML
- 1 tablespoon grated Parmesan cheese /15G
- 1 tablespoon olive oil /15ML
- 1/2 (10.75 ounces) can condensed cream of chicken soup /322.5ML
- 1/2 (10.75 ounces) can condensed cream of mushroom soup /322.5ML
- 1/2 cup dry bread crumbs /65G
- 1/2 cup dry fusilli pasta, cooked based on manufacturer's instructions /65G
- 1-1/2 teaspoons dried basil /7.5G
- 1-1/2 teaspoons dried minced onion /7.5G
- 1-1/2 teaspoons dried parsley /7.5G
- 3 chicken tenderloins, cut into chunks
- garlic powder to taste
- salt and pepper to taste

Instructions:

1) Grease baking pan of air fryer lightly with olive oil. Add chicken. Season with parsley, basil, garlic powder, pepper, salt, and minced onion.

2) Cook at 360° F or 183°C for 10 minutes. After 5 minutes stir the chicken to ensure even cooking.

3) Remove the basket, stir in mixed vegetables, cream of mushroom soup, cream of chicken soup, and cooked pasta. Mix well.

4) Mix melted butter, parmesan, and bread crumbs in a bowl. Evenly spread on the top of casserole.

5) Cook for 20 minutes at 390° F or 199°C .

6) Serve and enjoy.

Nutrition Information:

- Calories per Serving: 399
- Carbs: 35.4g
- Protein: 19.8g
- Fat: 19.8g

Chili, Lime & Corn Chicken BBQ

Servings per Recipe: 4

Cooking Time: 40 minutes

Ingredients:

- ½ teaspoon cumin /2.5G
- 1 tablespoon lime juice /15ML
- 1 teaspoon chili powder /5G
- 2 chicken breasts
- 2 chicken thighs
- 2 cups barbecue sauce /500ML
- 2 teaspoons grated lime zest /10G
- 4 ears of corn, cleaned
- Salt and pepper to taste

Instructions:

1) Place all ingredients inside a Ziploc bag except for the corn. Allow to marinate in the fridge for a couple of hours.
2) Preheat mid-air fryer to 390° F or 199°C .
3) Place the grill pan accessory inside the air fryer.
4) Grill the chicken and corn for 40 minutes.
5) Meanwhile, pour the marinade inside a saucepan over medium heat until it thickens.

6) Before serving, brush the chicken and corn with the sauce.

Nutrition information:

- Calories per serving: 849
- Carbs: 87.7g
- Protein: 52.3g
- Fat: 32.1g

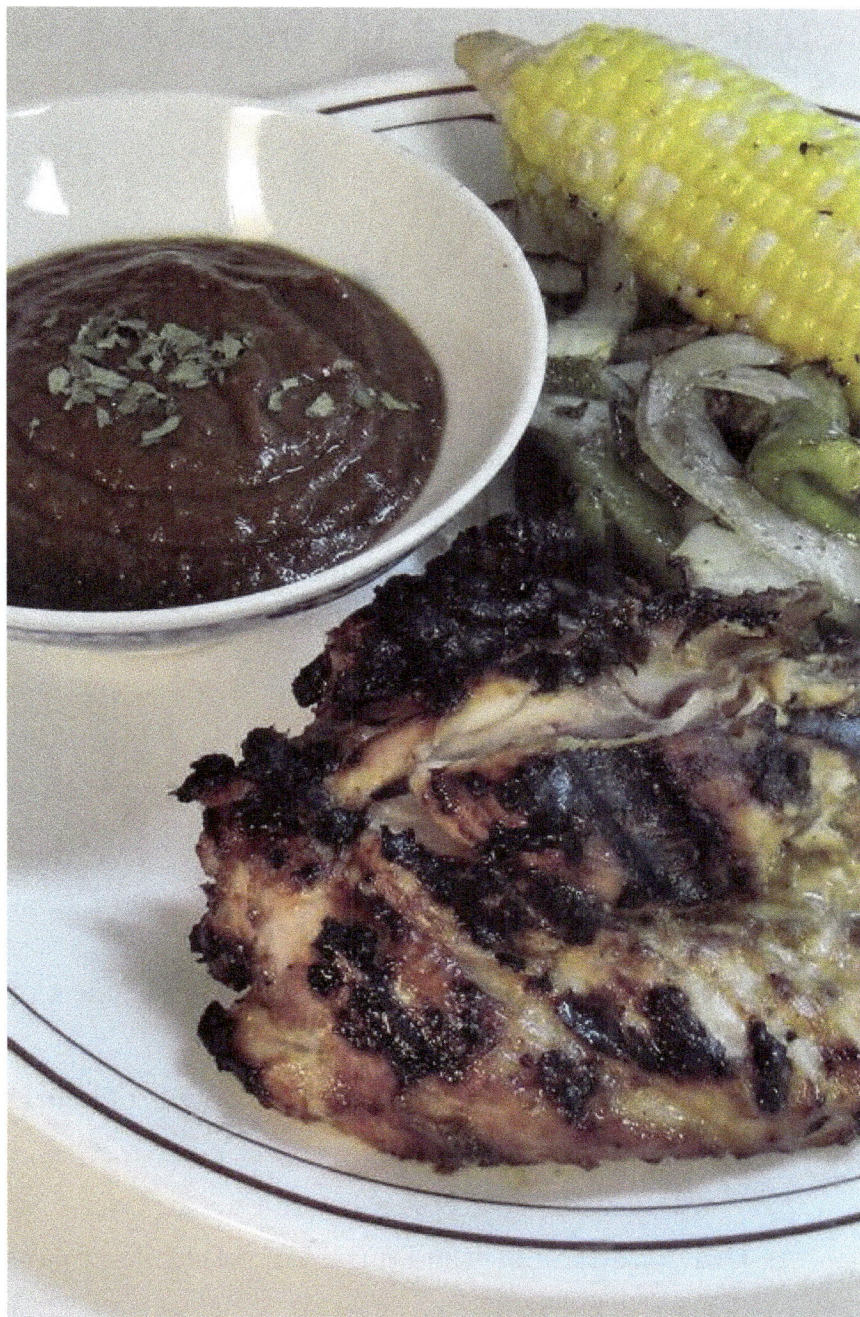

Chinese Five Spiced Marinated Chicken

Servings per Recipe: 4

Cooking Time: 40 minutes

Ingredients

- ¼ cup hoisin sauce /62.5ML
- 1 ¼ teaspoons sesame oil /6.25ML
- 1 ½ teaspoon five-spice powder /7.5G
- 2 chicken breasts, halved
- 2 tablespoons rice vinegar /30ML
- 2 teaspoons brown sugar /10G
- 3 ½ teaspoons grated ginger /17.5G
- 3 ½ teaspoons honey /17.5ML
- 3 cucumbers, sliced
- Salt and pepper to taste

Instructions:

1) Place all ingredients except the cucumber inside a Ziploc bag.
2) Allow to marinate in the fridge for a couple of hours.
3) Preheat air fryer to 390° F or 199°C .
4) Place the grill pan accessory within the air fryer.
5) Grill for 40 minutes and turn over the chicken frequently.
6) Serve chicken with cucumber once cooked.

Nutrition information:

- Calories per serving: 330
- Carbs:16.7 g
- Protein: 31.2g
- Fat: 15.4g

Chipotle Chicken ala King

Servings per Recipe: 4

Cooking Time: 40 minutes

Ingredients:

- 1 tablespoon sour cream /15ML
- 1 teaspoon ground cumin /5G
- 4 corn tortillas, cut into quarters
- 1/2 (10.75 ounces) can condensed cream of mushroom soup /322.5G
- 1/2 (10.75 ounces) can condensed cream of chicken soup /322.5G
- 1-1/2 teaspoons vegetable oil /7.5ML
- 1/2 white onion, diced
- 1/2 red bell pepper, diced
- 1/2 green bell pepper, diced
- 1/2 (10 ounces) can diced tomatoes with green chile peppers (including RO*TEL®) /300G
- 1/2 cup chicken broth /125ML
- 1/2 teaspoon ancho chile powder /2.5G
- 1/2 cooked chicken, torn into shreds or cut into chunks
- 1/4 teaspoon dried oregano /1.25G
- 1/4-pound shredded Cheddar cheese /1.25G
- 1/8 teaspoon chipotle chile powder /0.625G

Instructions:

1) Use vegetable oil to lightly grease the baking pan of the air fryer. Add bell pepper, red bell pepper, and onion. For 5 minutes, cook at 360° F or 183°C .

2) Add chipotle chile powder, oregano, ancho chile powder, cumin, sour cream, chicken broth, diced tomatoes, cream of chicken soup, and cream of mushroom soup in a large bowl and mix well.

3) Pour cooked sweet pepper into the bowl of sauce and mix well.

4) Add a few scoops of sauce to the bottom of the air fryer baking pan. Place ½ of chicken on top of the sauce, also top with 1/3 cheese, cover using a layer of corn tortilla. Repeat the process until all ingredients are used up.

5) Cover the pan with foil.

6) Cook for 25 minutes. Uncover and continue cooking for an additional 10 Minutes.

7) Serve and enjoy.

Nutrition Information:

- Calories per Serving: 482
- Carbs: 25.1g
- Protein: 32.1g
- Fat: 28.1g

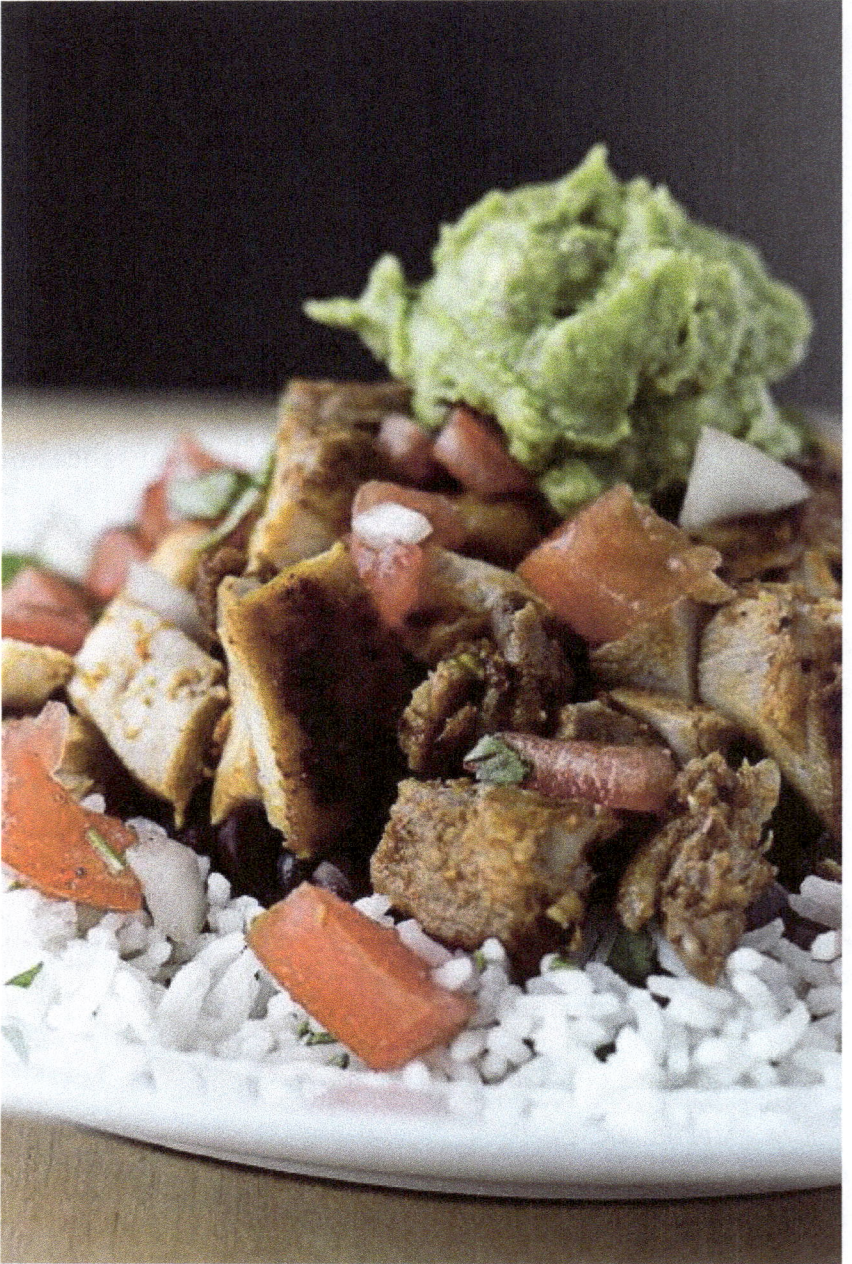

Honey-Balsamic Orange Chicken

Servings per Recipe: 3

Cooking Time: 40 minutes

Ingredients:

- ½ cup balsamic vinegar /125ML
- ½ cup honey /125ML
- 1 ½ pounds boneless chicken breasts, pounded /675G
- 1 tablespoon orange zest /15G
- 1 teaspoon fresh oregano, chopped /5G
- 2 tablespoons extra virgin olive oil /30ML
- Salt and pepper to taste

Instructions:

1) First put the chicken inside a Ziploc bag and add the other ingredients, shake well to combine. Place in the refrigerator for two hours.
2) Preheat the air fryer to 390° F or 199°C .
3) Place the grill pan in the air fryer.
4) Grill the chicken for 40 minutes.

Nutrition information:

- Calories per serving: 521
- Carbs: 56.1g
- Protein: 51.8g

- Fat: 9.9g

Lebanese Style Grilled Chicken

Servings per Recipe: 3

Cooking Time: 20 Minutes

Ingredients:

- 1 onion, cut into large chunks
- 1 small green bell pepper, cut into large chunks
- 1 teaspoon tomato paste /5ML
- 1/2 cup chopped fresh flat-leaf parsley /65G
- 1/2 teaspoon dried oregano /2.5G
- 1/3 cup plain yogurt /83ML
- 1/8 teaspoon ground allspice /0.625G
- 1/8 teaspoon ground black pepper /0.625G
- 1/8 teaspoon ground cardamom /0.625G
- 1/8 teaspoon ground cinnamon /0.625G
- 1-pound skinless, boneless chicken breast halves cut into 2-inch pieces /450G
- 2 cloves garlic, minced
- 2 tablespoons lemon juice /30ML
- 2 tablespoons vegetable oil /30ML
- 3/4 teaspoon salt /3.75G

Instructions:

1) Add cardamom, cinnamon, allspice, pepper, oregano, salt, tomato paste, garlic, yogurt, vegetable oil, and fresh lemon juice in a Ziploc bag. Add chicken, mix, press to remove excess air, seal, and marinate inside refrigerator for 4 hours.
2) Thread chicken into skewers, place on skewer rack and cook in batches.
3) For 10 minutes, cook on 360° F or 183°C . Turn over skewer after 5 minutes.
4) Serve with a sprinkle of parsley and enjoy.

Nutrition Information:

- Calories per Serving: 297
- Carbs: 9.8g
- Protein: 34.3g
- Fat: 13.4g

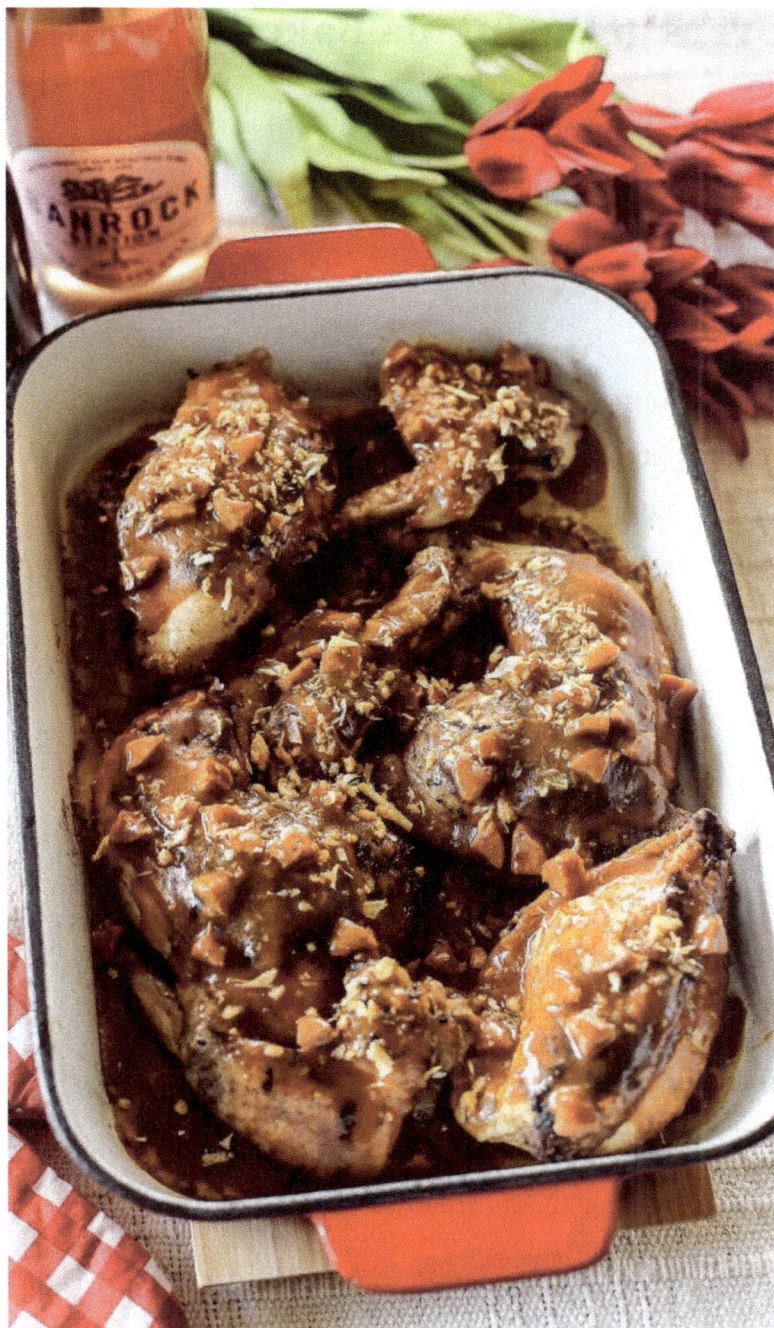

Leftovers 'n Enchilada Bake

Servings per Recipe: 3

Cooking Time: 45 minutes

Ingredients:

- 1 egg
- 1/2 (15 ounces) can black beans, drained /450G
- 1/2 (15 ounces) can tomato sauce /450ML
- 1/2 (7.5 ounces) package corn bread mix /225G
- 1/2 cup shredded Mexican-style cheese blend, or even more to taste /65G
- 1/2 envelope taco seasoning mix
- 1/2-pound chicken tenderloins /225G
- 1-1/2 teaspoons vegetable oil /7.5G
- 2 tablespoons cream cheese /30G
- 2 tablespoons water /30ML
- 2-1/4 teaspoons chili powder /11.25G
- 3 tablespoons milk /45ML

Instructions:

1) Oil baking pan. Add chicken and cook for 5 minutes at 360° F or 183°C .

2) While stirring add the chili powder, taco seasoning mix, water, and tomato sauce. Cook for 10 minutes, continue mixing and turning the chicken. Keep stirring and turning chicken halfway through cooking time.

3) Remove chicken from pan and shred with two forks. Return to pan and stir in cream cheese and black beans. Mix well.

4) Top with Mexican cheese.

5) Whisk egg and milk until thoroughly beaten. Add cornbread mix and mix well. Pour over chicken.

6) Cover pan with foil.

7) Cook for additional 15 minutes. Remove foil and cook for 10 more minutes or until topping is lightly browned.

8) Let it sit for 5 minutes.

9) Serve and enjoy.

Nutrition Information:

- Calories per Serving: 487
- Carbs: 45.9g
- Protein: 31.2g
- Fat: 19.8g

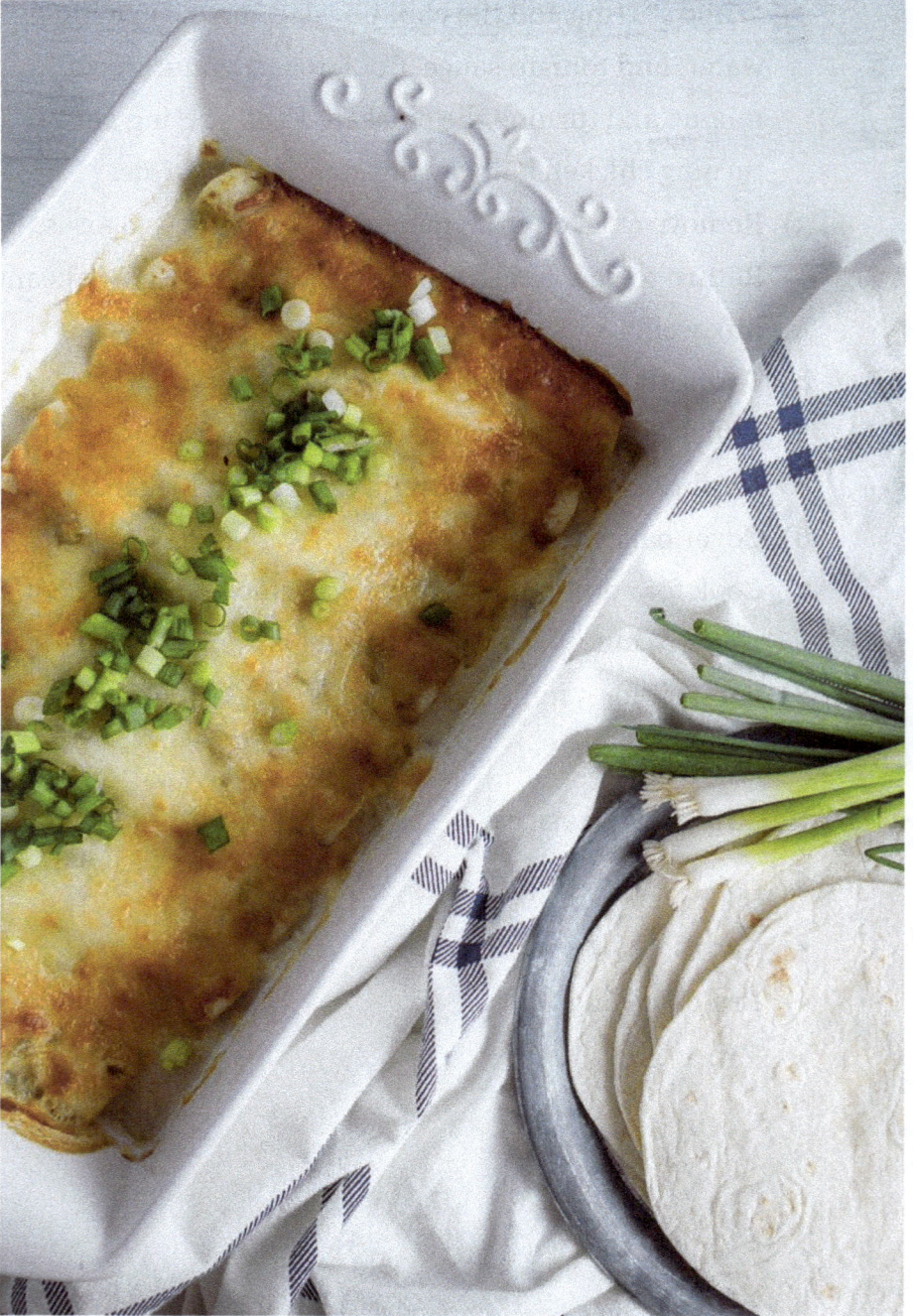

Lemon-Aleppo Chicken

Servings per Recipe: 4

Cooking Time: 1 hour

Ingredients

- ¼ cup Aleppo-style pepper /32.5G
- ¼ cup fresh lemon juice /62.5ML
- ¼ cup oregano /32.5G
- 1 cup green olives, pitted and cracked /130G
- 1.4 cups chopped rosemary /182G
- 2 pounds whole chicken, backbones removed and butterflied /900G
- 6 cloves of garlic, minced
- Salt and pepper to taste

Instructions:

1) Place the chicken side up and slice the breasts. Press your hand against the breast bone to flatten the breast tissue or remove the bones altogether.
2) Season the boneless chicken with salt, pepper, garlic, pepper, rosemary, lemon juice, and oregano.
3) Allow to marinate inside the fridge for at least 12 hours.
4) Preheat the air fryer to 390° F or 199°C .
5) Place the grill pan accessory in the air fryer.

6) Place the chicken on the grill pan and place the olives across the chicken.

7) Grill for 1 hour and turn over the chicken every 10 minutes for even grilling.

Nutrition information:

- Calories per serving: 502
- Carbs:50.4 g
- Protein:37.6 g
- Fat: 16.6g

Blueberry & Lemon Cake

Servings per Recipe: 4

Cooking Time: 17 minutes

Ingredients:

- 2 eggs
- 1 cup blueberries /130G
- zest from 1 lemon
- juice from 1 lemon
- 1 tsp. vanilla /5ML
- brown sugar for topping (somewhat sprinkling together with each muffin-less than a teaspoon)
- 2 1/2 cups self-rising flour /325G
- 1/2 cup Monk Fruit (or use your preferred sugar) /65G
- 1/2 cup cream /125ML
- 1/4 cup avocado oil (any light cooking oil) /62.5ML

Instructions:

1) Place all ingredients in a mixing bowl and mix. Add the dry ingredients and mix well.
2) Grease baking pan lightly with oil using cooking spray. Pour the batter in.
3) Cook at 330° F or 166°C for 12 minutes.
4) Let it stay at home air fryer for 5 minutes.
5) Serve, eat and enjoy.

Nutrition Information:

- Calories per Serving: 589
- Carbs: 76.7g
- Protein: 13.5g
- Fat: 25.3g

Bread Pudding with Cranberry

Servings per Recipe: 4

Cooking Time: 45 minutes

Ingredients:

- 1-1/2 cups milk /375ML
- 2-1/2 eggs
- 1/2 cup cranberries1 teaspoon butter /70G
- 1/4 cup and two tablespoons white sugar /62.5G
- 1/4 cup golden raisins /32.5G
- 1/8 teaspoon ground cinnamon /0.625G
- 3/4 cup heavy whipping cream /188ML
- 3/4 teaspoon lemon zest /3.75G
- 3/4 teaspoon kosher salt /3.75G
- 3/4 French baguettes, cut into 2-inch slices
- 3/8 vanilla bean, split and seeds scraped away

Instructions:

1) Grease baking pan with oil. Spread baguette slices, cranberries, and raisins in the pan.
2) Blend vanilla bean, cinnamon, salt, lemon zest, eggs, sugar, and cream. Pour this mixture over baguette slices. Let it soak for an hour.
3) Cover pan with foil.
4) Cook for 35 minutes at 330° F or 166°C .

5) Let it sit for 10 minutes.

6) Serve and enjoy

Nutrition Information:

- Calories per Serving: 581
- Carbs: 76.1g
- Protein: 15.8g
- Fat: 23.7g

Cherries 'n Almond Flour Bars

Serves: 12

Cooking Time: 35 minutes

Ingredients

- ¼ cup water /62.5ML
- ½ cup butter softened /65G
- ½ teaspoon salt / 2.5G
- ½ teaspoon vanilla /2.5G
- 1 ½ cups almond flour /195G
- 1 cup erythritol /130G
- 1 cup fresh cherries, pitted /130G
- 1 tablespoon xanthan gum /15G
- 2 eggs

Instructions:

1) Add the first 6 ingredients to a mixing bowl, mix well to form a dough.
2) Add the dough to the baking pan.
3) Place in the air fryer and bake for 10 minutes at 375° F or 191°C .
4) Meanwhile, mix the cherries, water, and xanthan gum in a bowl.
5) Take the dough out and pour on the cherry mixture.

6) Return the baking pan to the mid-air fryer and cook again for 25 minutes at 375° F or 191°C .

Nutrition information:

- Calories per serving: 99
- Carbohydrates: 2.1g
- Protein: 1.8g
- Fat: 9.3g

Cherry-Choco Bars

Serves: 8

Cooking Time: 15

Ingredients:

- ¼ teaspoon salt /1.25G
- ½ cup almonds, sliced /65G
- ½ cup chia seeds /65G
- ½ cup chocolate brown, chopped /65G
- ½ cup dried cherries, chopped /65G
- ½ cup prunes, pureed /65G
- ½ cup quinoa, cooked /65G
- ¾ cup almond butter /98G
- 1/3 cup honey /83ML
- 2 cups old-fashioned oats /260G
- 2 tablespoon coconut oil /30ML

Instructions:

1) Preheat mid-air fryer to 375° F or 191°C .
2) Add the oats, quinoa, chia seeds, almond, cherries, and chocolate to a mixing bowl, mix well to combine.
3) Heat the almond butter, honey, and coconut oil.
4) Pour the butter mixture into the dry mixture. Add salt and prunes.
5) Mix until well combined.

6) Pour the mixture into the baking dish.

7) Cook for 15 minutes.

8) Let it cool for an hour before slicing it into bars.

Nutrition information:

- Calories per serving: 321

- Carbohydrates: 35g

- Protein: 7g

- Fat: 17g

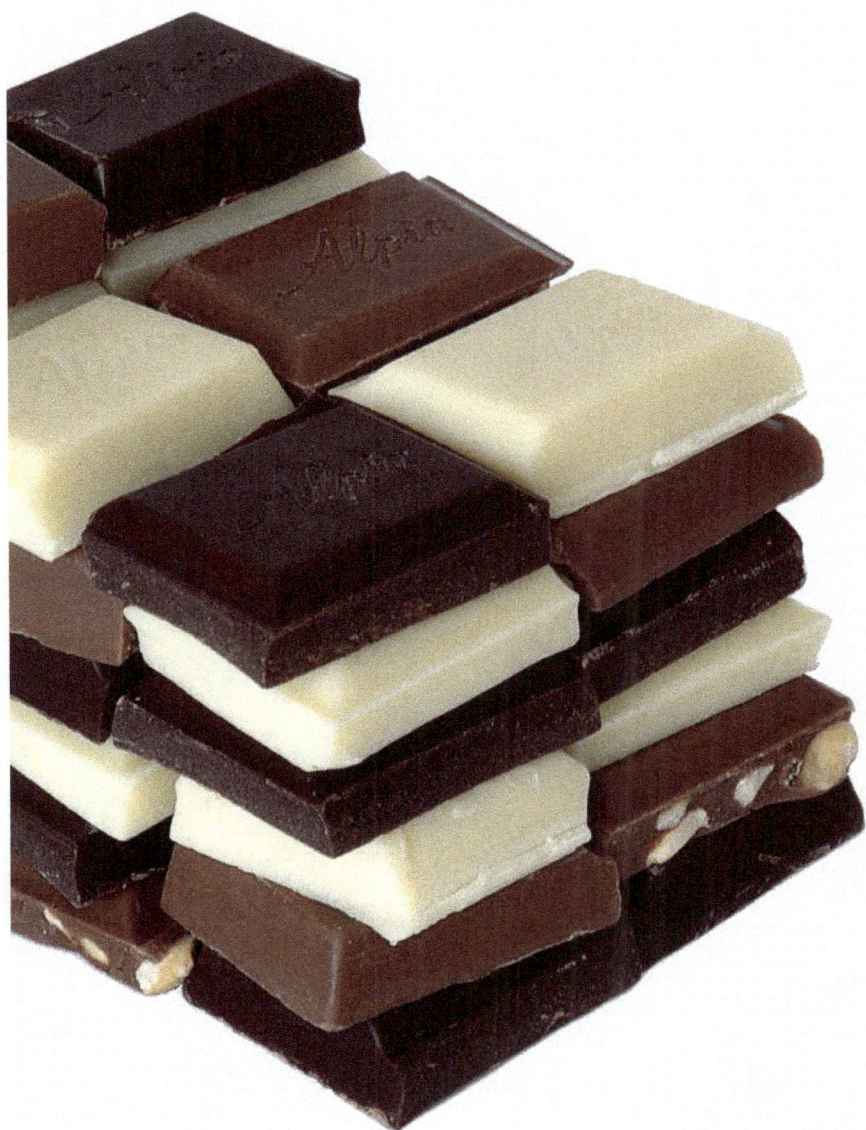

www.ingramcontent.com/pod-product-compliance
Lightning Source LLC
Chambersburg PA
CBHW062117040426
42336CB00041B/1661